VITAMINS AND MINERALS

SUPPLEMENTS FOR WELLNESS AND LONGEVITY

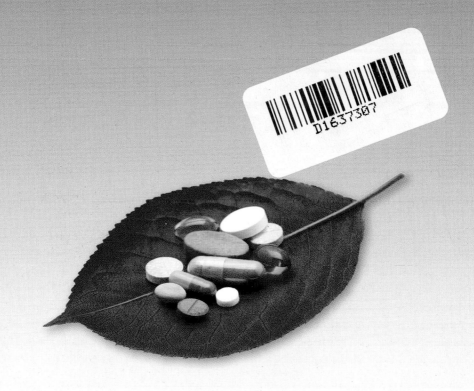

Publications International, Ltd.

Written by: Susan Male Smith, M.A., R.D., Arline McDonald, Ph.D., Densie Webb, Ph.D., R.D., Annette Natow, Ph.D., R.D., and Jo-Ann Heslin, M.A., R.D.

Photography: Shutterstock.com and Wikimedia Commons

All Dietary Reference Intake tables from Institute of Medicine. Washington, DC: The National Academies Press.

All Food Sources tables from National Institute of Health, Office of Dietary Supplements.

ISBN: 978-1-64030-594-6

Manufactured in China.

8 7 6 5 4 3 2 1

Let's get social!
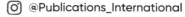
@Publications_International
@PublicationsInternational
www.pilbooks.com

Table of Contents

Introduction

Throughout most of history, no one knew vitamins or minerals existed—at least, not by name. People knew only the results of not having certain foods in their diets.

Deciding what to eat back then was relatively simple. You ate whatever food was around. If you were lucky, nutrients balanced themselves in the available food, keeping you and your neighbors healthy. But at times, inevitably, the diet lacked various essential nutrients, and the entire population suffered the consequences. By trial and error, people improved their diets, recognizing in some elementary way the connection between good food and good health.

Today, we have a wealth of knowledge about essential nutrients. We know what each nutrient does for us when taken in normal amounts, as well as effects they may have when taken in large doses. Now we have a new problem—too much information. There are so many reports about vitamins, minerals, and supplements—which should we believe?

We've cut through the confusion and have come up with a clear explanation of the function, value, and potential benefits of each nutrient. We emphasize throughout that you should meet recommended nutrient intakes by eating a balanced diet. It's our hope that the information in this book will compel you to select foods that will contribute to a healthier life.

CHAPTER 1
The Fundamentals of Nutrition

Studying only vitamins and minerals in the school of nutrition is like studying only verbs and nouns in an English class—they're only part of the overall picture. We must also understand what other elements food contains, why we need them, and how they're used in our bodies. Once we understand the intricate workings of essential nutrients, we'll have the knowledge we need to eat better and live a healthier life.

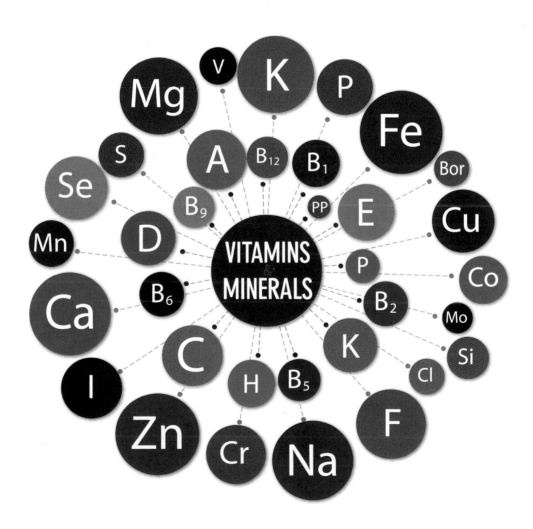

History

About 10,000 years ago, people developed agriculture. They began to farm and domesticate animals, thereby working with the environment to take care of themselves. From ignorance evolved curiosity about how food sustains life. With the dawning of the scientific age, people began to ask more questions: What happens to food when it's eaten? How does food generate energy? What foods are important for growth and the maintenance of health? These and other questions remained unanswered until chemistry, biochemistry, physiology, and other related sciences advanced.

In the late 1700s, Antoine-Laurent Lavoisier (*right*), a French nobleman often considered the "father of modern chemistry," investigated the relationship between respiration and energy production. His studies showed that our bodies use the oxygen we inhale to produce body heat and energy. He also observed that carbon dioxide is created and exhaled in the process. Lavoisier concluded that food acts as fuel, which the body oxidizes, or burns up, to release energy.

In a coal furnace, for example, coal burns in the presence of oxygen, releasing carbon dioxide and energy as heat. The oxidation of food is similar: In the presence of oxygen, the food we eat is burned to release carbon dioxide and energy. Lavoisier's work was the first step toward uncovering how food sustains life. But the oxidation of food is only a part of a complex series of reactions that occur in the body—reactions we refer to as metabolism.

Metabolism and Energy

Metabolism encompasses all the chemical reactions that take place in the body's trillions of cells. Our cells break down the molecules of some substances and build up the molecules of others. These chemical reactions are necessary to produce proteins, hormones, enzymes, fats, and stored forms of sugar that are vital to life. The reactions also produce energy, which is either stored or released.

Energy is simply the ability to do work. We get energy from burning food as fuel, and we can determine how much energy a certain food supplies. We talk about the energy value of foods by comparing the number of calories foods provide. A calorie is a unit of heat energy. The energy value of individual foods depends on the amount of carbohydrates, fats, and proteins present. Carbohydrates and proteins supply four calories per gram, while fats yield nine calories per gram. (One gram is about equal to the mass of a paper clip. For comparison to more meaningful measures: There are 28.3 grams in an ounce and 453.5 grams in a pound. A milligram [mg] is one thousandth of a gram; a microgram [mcg or µg] is one millionth of a gram, or one thousandth of a milligram.)

Different types of energy are interchangeable. For example, the chemical energy of carbohydrates, which are important body fuels, can be converted into heat energy to help maintain a constant body temperature. It can also change to kinetic energy necessary for muscle action, or it can be trapped as chemical energy and stored in other body compounds.

The Essential Nutrients

As the science of chemistry developed in the 18th and 19th centuries, so did procedures to analyze what we eat. Scientists soon discovered the great variety of chemically distinct compounds in foods. Their experiments determined which parts of foods are best suited for growth and health.

The English physician William Prout *(right)* was probably among the first to define an "adequate diet." In 1827, he described the three "staminal principles" of foods necessary to support life, which we know now as fats, carbohydrates, and proteins.

The study of food chemistry became increasingly sophisticated. By the latter part of the 19th century, the definition of Prout's "adequate diet" was expanded to include minerals.

But something was still missing. By the dawn of the 20th century, scientists found that experimental animals perished when fed diets containing only highly purified preparations of fats, carbohydrates, proteins, and the known minerals. The missing vital nutrients turned out to be vitamins, the fifth class of nutrients discovered. (Previous researchers had failed to recognize the existence of vitamins because the diets prepared for experimental animals were not sufficiently "pure"—they were "contaminated" with vitamins.) Today we recognize six classes of essential nutrients: carbohydrates, fats and oils (fatty acids), proteins (amino acids), vitamins, minerals, and water.

Classes of Essential Nutrients

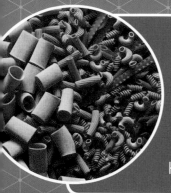

1. CARBOHYDRATES (STARCHES; SUGARS)

Carbohydrates are the body's primary source of fuel. Complex carbohydrates, found in grains, legumes, and starchy vegetables, provide vitamins, minerals, and fiber. Sugars, also known as simple carbohydrates, provide calories (and energy) with few nutrients. Carbohydrates provide four calories per gram.

2. FATS AND OILS (FATTY ACIDS)

Also called lipids; used to supply energy. Dietary fat supplies the two essential fatty acids, important components of cells that the body cannot synthesize. A layer of fat under the skin insulates the body. Fat around internal organs cushions and protects them. Accumulation of too much fat leads to being overweight or obese. Saturated fats, found in butter, stick margarine, meat, poultry skin, and whole-fat dairy foods, are solid at room temperature and can raise blood cholesterol levels. Unsaturated fats, found in vegetable oils, nuts, olives, and avocados, are liquid at room temperature and help lower blood cholesterol levels. Fat provides nine calories per gram.

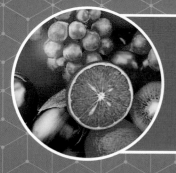

3. VITAMINS

Regulators of metabolism necessary for normal formation and breakdown of body carbohydrates, fats, and proteins. Many vitamins play roles as coenzymes, helping to trigger important reactions.

4. PROTEINS (AMINO ACIDS)

Used primarily in the growth and maintenance of lean body tissues—muscle. If necessary, our bodies use proteins for energy. Proteins are made up of smaller units called amino acids—nine of which are essential and must come from food. Animal sources of protein include fish, poultry, and meat. Plant sources include beans, nuts, and whole grains. Protein provides four calories per gram.

5. MINERALS

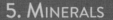

Also called inorganic elements; used for various functions. Minerals like calcium and phosphorus contribute to body structure as an important part of bones. Iron is a part of hemoglobin, the red pigment in blood that transports oxygen from the lungs to body tissues. Some inorganic elements are essential for optimal nerve and muscle response to stimuli. Others are essential for normal enzyme action.

6. WATER

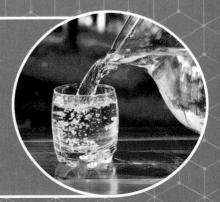

A component of every cell in the body, accounting for 60% of body weight. Water carries nutrients to cells and waste products away from them. Water also regulates body temperature, aids digestion, and acts as a lubricant and shock absorber.

Eating for Better Health

Although there are many guidelines for healthy eating, the simplest and most comprehensive are what are known as the *Dietary Guidelines for Americans*, which are revised and published every five years by the U.S. Departments of Agriculture (USDA) and Health and Human Services (HHS). The *Guidelines* provide food recommendations with the intention of promoting health, preventing chronic diseases, and helping people reach and maintain a healthy weight. They also serve as the basis of federal nutrition policy and programs.

The current *Dietary Guidelines for Americans* (2015–2020 edition) focus on healthy eating patterns as a whole, rather than individual foods or nutrients in isolation. That's because a growing body of research suggests that eating patterns may be more predictive of overall health status and disease risk than individual foods or nutrients.

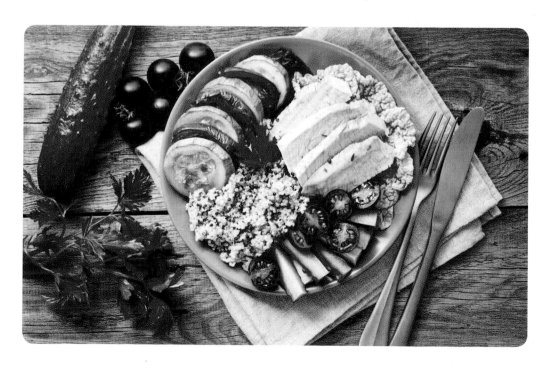

Healthy Eating Patterns

Your eating pattern represents the entirety of all foods and beverages you consume over time. To build a healthy eating pattern, choose a variety of nutritious foods in the right amounts for you—and make these choices part of your daily routine. Follow these tips—based on the *2015–2020 Dietary Guidelines for Americans*—that can help you reach or maintain a healthy body weight, get the nutrients you need, and lower your risk of health problems like heart disease, type 2 diabetes, and some types of cancers.

What a healthy eating pattern *includes*:

- A variety of vegetables from all subgroups—dark green, red and orange, starchy, legumes, and other vegetables
- Fruits, especially whole fruits
- Grains, at least half of which are whole grains
- Fat-free or low-fat dairy, including milk, yogurt, cheese, and fortified soy beverages
- A variety of protein foods, including seafood, lean meats and poultry, eggs, legumes, nuts, seeds, and soy products
- Oils

What a healthy eating pattern *limits*:

- Saturated fats and trans fats, added sugars, and sodium

Aim to consume:

- Less than 10% of calories each day from added sugars
- Less than 10% of calories each day from saturated fats
- Less than 2,300 milligrams of sodium each day for adults and children ages 14+ (less for younger children)

MyPlate

For more than a century, the U.S. Department of Agriculture (USDA) has provided dietary guidance to help Americans plan and evaluate their diets for adequate nutrition. The USDA's current food guide for consumers is MyPlate, which

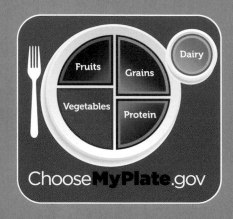

replaced earlier food pyramids. MyPlate illustrates the five food groups with the visual of a place setting. Because consumers have different calorie and nutrient needs, the MyPlate icon is suggestive of the relative proportions of food groups in the diet. For example, vegetables and fruits should fill half of your plate. ChooseMyPlate.gov provides resources based on the *2015–2020 Dietary Guidelines for Americans* to help people meet food group, nutrient, and calorie needs and make positive eating choices. These resources include a personalized MyPlate Plan, which shows you what and how much to eat within your calorie allowance based on your age, gender, height, weight, and physical activity level.

A Closer Look at Food Groups

Foods are grouped according to the nutrients they share. The five food groups are defined as vegetables, fruits, grains, dairy, and protein foods. Some of these food groups, including vegetables and grains, are divided into subgroups. Foods within a larger group are separated into subgroups based on their similarity in nutritional composition and other dietary benefits. Eating a variety of different nutrient-dense foods from across all groups and subgroups—in appropriate amounts—is the best way to meet nutrient needs. (Nutrient-dense foods provide nutrients and other beneficial substances with little or no solid fats and added sugars, refined starches, and sodium.)

Vegetables

Foods in this group are divided into five subgroups—dark green, red and orange, legumes (beans and peas), starchy, and other vegetables. Vegetables provide many nutrients, including dietary fiber, potassium, vitamins A, B_6, C, E, and K, copper, magnesium, folate, iron, manganese, thiamin, niacin, and choline. The best way to ensure you're getting the full benefits is to eat a variety of colorful vegetables from across all of the subgroups.

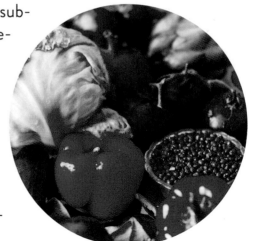

- **Dark green vegetables:** Broccoli, collard greens, kale, mustard greens, romaine lettuce, spinach, and turnip greens.
- **Red and orange vegetables:** Carrots, pumpkin, red peppers, sweet potatoes, tomatoes, tomato juice, and winter squash.

- **Legumes:** Black beans, chickpeas, edamame (green soybeans), kidney beans, lentils, pinto beans, split peas, and white beans. Does *not* include green (string) beans or green peas because their nutrient compositions are not similar to legumes.

- **Starchy vegetables:** Cassava, corn, green lima beans, green peas, plantains, and white potatoes.

- **Other vegetables:** Cabbage, celery, cucumbers, green (string) beans, green peppers, iceberg lettuce, mushrooms, onions, and zucchini.

Fruits

Foods in this group include all fresh, frozen, canned, and dried fruits and fruit juices. Dietary fiber, folate, potassium, and vitamin C are among the many nutrients fruits provide. Most fruits are naturally low in fat and calories, none have cholesterol, and many are great sources of fiber. To maximize the benefits of dietary fiber, focus on whole or cut-up fruit rather than juice. When selecting fruit juice, pick options that are 100% juice, without added sugars. When picking canned fruit, select fruit canned in water or 100% fruit juice rather than syrup.

Grains

The grains food group includes grains as single foods (e.g., oatmeal, rice, popcorn), as well as products that include grains as an ingredient (e.g., breads, crackers, cereals, and pasta). Grain-based foods are rich in complex carbohydrates, your body's best energy source.

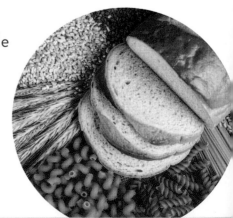

As the body's key fuel, carbohydrates provide your brain, heart, and nervous system with a constant supply of energy to keep you moving, breathing, and thinking.

Grain products also supply B vitamins and iron (especially if they're enriched or include the whole grain), as well as other beneficial phytonutrients (substances in plants with health-protective effects). In addition, many grain-based foods supply fiber.

Grains are either whole or refined. Whole grains supply nutrients such as iron, zinc, manganese, folate, magnesium, copper, thiamin, niacin, phosphorus, selenium, riboflavin, vitamin A, and vitamin B_6. Whole grains contain the entire kernel, including the endosperm, bran, and germ. Refined grains have been processed to remove the bran and germ.

The Whole Story

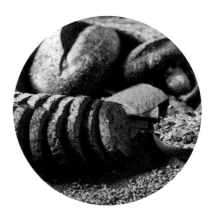

An important strategy for choosing the best grain foods is to seek out products made from whole grains. A whole grain is the entire edible part of any grain, whether it's wheat, oats, corn, rice, or a more exotic grain. The three layers of a grain kernel each supply important nutrients:

- The outer protective coating, or bran, is packed with fiber, B vitamins, protein, and trace minerals.
- The endosperm supplies mostly carbohydrate and protein and some B vitamins.
- The germ is rich in B vitamins, vitamin E, trace minerals, antioxidants, and phytonutrients.

When whole grains are milled (refined), the bran and the germ portions are removed, leaving only the endosperm. Unfortunately, more than half the fiber and almost three-quarters of the vitamins and minerals are in the bran and germ. When you eat foods made from whole grains, you get the nutritional benefits of the entire grain. Most refined grains are enriched. Enriched grain products add back some of the B vitamins—thiamin, folic acid, riboflavin, and niacin—and iron lost when the grain was milled. But lots of other nutrients and fiber don't get added back.

A diet rich in whole-grain foods is associated with lower risk for several chronic diseases and conditions including heart disease, cancer, diabetes, and gastrointestinal troubles. It can also play a role in the treatment of many of these diseases.

Dairy

Dairy foods include yogurt, cheese, milk (including lactose-free and lactose-reduced products), and fortified soy beverages (soymilk). Foods in the dairy group supply approximately 75 percent of the calcium we consume. In addition, they provide protein, phosphorus, magnesium, and vitamins A, D, B_{12}, riboflavin, potassium, zinc, choline, and selenium. Although milk, yogurt, and cheese offer significant amounts of calcium and other key nutrients, most people eat only half the recommended daily servings from this group. (And note that teens require more calcium than adults.) That means many people—adults and children—may not be getting enough calcium and other nutrients essential to staying healthy. Certainly, foods from other groups contain calcium, but foods outside this group generally contain less, and the body may not absorb it as well.

Also note: Other dairy-based foods, such as butter, cream cheese, and sour cream, are not considered dairy servings. These foods are made from the cream portion of milk and contain mostly fat and little, if any, calcium.

Protein Foods

The diverse foods in this group have something important in common—protein. The amount and quality of the protein in these foods vary, but all are considered high-protein foods. The animal foods contain high-quality, or complete, proteins, which means they supply all the amino acids your body needs to build the proteins used to support body functions. The plant sources of protein supply lesser amounts, and the proteins are not complete; all of the amino acids are not found in a single source, although plant sources can be combined to provide the amino acids needed to form complete proteins.

Besides protein, foods from this group supply varying amounts of other nutrients, including iron, selenium, choline, phosphorus, zinc, copper, vitamin D, vitamin E, and B vitamins (thiamin, niacin, and vitamins B_6 and B_{12}). On the downside, some of the foods in this group contain higher amounts of fat and saturated fat. Some also include cholesterol.

Dietary Reference Intakes (DRIs)

Dietary Reference Intakes (DRIs) are a set of reference values for specific nutrients. These values are used to plan and evaluate nutrient intakes of healthy people. For each essential nutrient, a committee of experts reviews the latest scientific evidence to help inform standards of adequacy and toxicity for groups of people of different genders and at different life stages.

The DRIs expand on the Recommended Dietary Allowances (RDAs), which were issued periodically from 1941 to 1989 by the National Academy of Sciences. The Recommended Dietary Allowances were an outgrowth of the need to determine the U.S. population's food and nutrition status as it related to national defense during World War II. The productivity of the American people depended on good health, and good health depended on good nutrition.

The very first report of Recommended Dietary Allowances, published in 1941, recommended intakes for calories, protein, and the 8 vitamins and minerals deemed most important. By 1989, the report gave RDAs for 11 vitamins, 7 minerals, and protein, plus "estimated safe and adequate daily dietary intakes" for 7 additional vitamins and minerals. DRIs now cover more than 40 nutrient substances. (For recommended intakes, see individual nutrient profiles in Chapter 6.)

Key Terms

DIETARY REFERENCE INTAKES (DRIs)

A set of nutrient-based reference values that are quantitative estimates of nutrient intakes to be used for planning and assessing diets for healthy people. This umbrella term includes Estimated Average Requirement (EAR), Recommended Dietary Allowance (RDA), Adequate Intake (AI), and Tolerable Upper Intake Level (UL).

RECOMMENDED DIETARY ALLOWANCES (RDAs)

The average daily intake level sufficient to meet the nutrient requirements of nearly all (97–98%) healthy people in a particular group.

ESTIMATED AVERAGE REQUIREMENTS (EARs)

The average daily intake level estimated to meet the nutrient requirements of half the healthy people in a particular group. Used to calculate the RDA.

ADEQUATE INTAKES (AIs)

The recommended daily intake of a nutrient believed to ensure nutritional adequacy in most people. Used when evidence is insufficient to develop an RDA.

TOLERABLE UPPER INTAKE LEVELS (ULs)

The maximum average daily nutrient intake level unlikely to cause adverse health effects for most people in a particular group. As intake increases above the UL, the risk of adverse health effects increases.

Nutrition Labeling

The Nutrition Facts Label on packaged foods and beverages can help consumers learn about and compare the nutrient content of foods. The Percent Daily Value (% Daily Value or %DV) on the Nutrition Facts Label shows how much of a nutrient is in one serving, and how that contributes to a total daily diet. The %DV is based on the Daily Value (DV) for key nutrients. Daily Values are reference amounts (in grams, milligrams, or micrograms) of nutrients recommended per day for Americans four years of age and older.

The U.S. Food and Drug Administration (FDA) announced a new Nutrition Facts Label in May 2016 for packaged foods. The new label reflects updated scientific information, including the link between diet and chronic diseases. Below are some of the key changes to the Nutrition Facts Label.

• The number of "servings per container" and the "Serving size" declaration have increased and are now in larger and/or bolder type. Serving sizes have been updated to reflect what people actually consume today, rather than a recommendation of how much to consume.

OLD LABEL

Nutrition Facts
Serving Size 2/3 cup (55g)
Servings Per Container About 8

Amount Per Serving

Calories 230	Calories from Fat 40

	% Daily Value*
Total Fat 8g	12%
Saturated Fat 1g	5%
Trans Fat 0g	
Cholesterol 0mg	0%
Sodium 160mg	7%
Total Carbohydrate 37g	12%
Dietary Fiber 4g	16%
Sugars 1g	
Protein 3g	

Vitamin A	10%
Vitamin C	8%
Calcium	20%
Iron	45%

* Percent Daily Values are based on a 2,000 calorie diet. Your daily value may be higher or lower depending on your calorie needs.

	Calories:	2,000	2,500
Total Fat	Less than	65g	80g
Sat Fat	Less than	20g	25g
Cholesterol	Less than	300mg	300mg
Sodium	Less than	2,400mg	2,400mg
Total Carbohydrate		300g	375g
Dietary Fiber		25g	30g

NEW LABEL

Nutrition Facts
8 servings per container
Serving size   2/3 cup (55g)

Amount per serving

Calories   230

	% Daily Value*
Total Fat 8g	10%
Saturated Fat 1g	5%
Trans Fat 0g	
Cholesterol 0mg	0%
Sodium 160mg	7%
Total Carbohydrate 37g	13%
Dietary Fiber 4g	14%
Total Sugars 12g	
Includes 10g Added Sugars	20%
Protein 3g	

Vitamin D 2mcg	10%
Calcium 260mg	20%
Iron 8mg	45%
Potassium 235mg	6%

* The % Daily Value (DV) tells you how much a nutrient in a serving of food contributes to a daily diet. 2,000 calories a day is used for general nutrition advice.

- "Calories" is now larger and bolder. "Calories from Fat" has been removed because research shows the type of fat consumed is more important than the amount.

- "Added Sugars" in grams and as a %DV is now required. Scientific data shows that it's difficult to meet nutrient needs while staying within calorie limits if you consume more than 10 percent of your total daily calories from added sugar.

- The list of nutrients that are required or permitted on the label has been updated. Vitamin D and potassium are now required. Vitamins A and C are no longer required but can be included voluntarily. Vitamin D, calcium, iron, and potassium must be listed in milligrams or micrograms in addition to the %DV.

Key Terms

DAILY VALUE (DV)
The amount of a nutrient recommended per day for adults and children ages 4 and up. The U.S. Food and Drug Administration (FDA) establishes Daily Values. The Daily Values are used to calculate the Percent Daily Value (%DV) that manufacturers include on the label.

PERCENT DAILY VALUE (%DV)
The percentage of the Daily Value (the amounts of nutrients recommended per day) for each nutrient in one serving of the food. The %DV on the label helps consumers understand the nutrition information in the context of a total daily diet.

CHAPTER 2
Vitamins

Vitamins are organic substances that are necessary in very small amounts to maintain normal metabolism in the body.

In 1912, Dr. Casimir Funk *(right)*, a Polish chemist working at the Lister Institute in London, coined the word *vitamine*. He derived it from *vita*, meaning "life," and *amine*, referring to a class of nitrogen-containing organic compounds. At the time, Dr. Funk was investigating thiamin—vitamin B_1—which is an amine. Later, scientists realized that not all vitamins are amines, so the final *e* in *vitamine* was dropped. The word vitamin reflects the vital life-giving importance of these substances.

The phrase "in very small amounts" included in the definition of vitamins sets them apart from the other classes of essential organic compounds. For example, proteins, fats, and carbohydrates are also organic substances, but we require them in considerably greater quantities. We measure vitamins in milligrams (mg) and micrograms (mcg or μg); in contrast, we measure proteins, fats, and carbohydrates in grams (g).

We've only known about the existence of vitamins since Dr. Funk's research in 1912. Since that time, scientists have identified approximately 13 vitamins. The last to be isolated was vitamin B_{12} in the late 1940s. Upon its discovery, researchers assigned a letter designation to each vitamin in alphabetical order. It turned out, however, that some of the vitamins were actually several substances. The compound vitamin B, for example, turned out to be a group of compounds. So we now have vitamin B_1, vitamin B_2, vitamin B_6, and so forth. Although vitamins' alphabetical designations are still in common use, they also have chemical names. (The table below identifies the 13 vitamins and their chemical names.)

VITAMIN	CHEMICAL NAME(S)
Vitamin A	Beta-carotene; retinol
Vitamin B_1	Thiamine
Vitamin B_2	Riboflavin
Vitamin B_3	Niacin; niacinamide
Vitamin B_5	Pantothenic acid
Vitamin B_6	Pyridoxine; pyridoxamine; pyridoxal
Vitamin B_7	Biotin
Vitamin B_9	Folic acid; folate
Vitamin B_{12}	Cobalamin; cyanocobalamin; hydroxycobalamin; methylcobalamin
Vitamin C	Ascorbic acid
Vitamin D	Cholecalciferol (D_3); ergocalciferol (D_2)
Vitamin E	Tocopherol; tocotrienols
Vitamin K	Menadione (K_3); menaquinone (K_2); phylloquinone, phytomenadione, phytonadione (K_1)

All vitamins are essential to life and must be supplied in the diet. As with any rule, though, there are exceptions. The body does produce small amounts of biotin, vitamin B_{12}, and vitamin K from intestinal bacteria, but in such negligible quantities that we still need more from the foods we eat.

Furthermore, if the body is supplied with the proper raw materials, it is capable of manufacturing certain other vitamins. For example, plant foods such as fruits and vegetables don't actually contain vitamin A but instead have vitamin A "activity." In other words, they are "precursors" to vitamin A because they contain substances called carotenes that our bodies can convert to vitamin A. Carotenoid is the substance that makes certain fruits and vegetables yellow, orange, or red. Some carotenoids, such as beta-carotene, alpha-carotene, and beta-cryptoxanthin, can be made into vitamin A by the body. Other carotenoids, such as lycopene, lutein, and zeaxanthin, cannot be made into vitamin A by the body. All carotenoids are antioxidants. These precursors are sometimes called provitamin A. Carotenes may also function as antioxidants, giving them importance beyond their conversion to vitamin A. (See Chapter 4 for more on antioxidants.)

We have a provitamin D in our skin. Sunlight triggers a chemical reaction in skin that begins the provitamin's complex conversion to vitamin D—a process that is later completed in the kidneys. This explains vitamin D's nickname, the "sunshine vitamin." Often, though, the amount produced this way isn't enough to meet our bodies' needs, and we still need a dietary source.

The body also meets some of its niacin needs by conversion from the amino acid tryptophan. Because we must rely on diet to fulfill our requirements for these vitamins, they are all essential.

Water-Soluble vs. Fat-Soluble Vitamins

One way to classify vitamins is by solubility. Water-soluble vitamins—the B vitamins and vitamin C—dissolve in water. Water-soluble vitamins can't be stored in the body, so you need them more frequently. Excess vitamins are excreted in urine. Water-soluble vitamins are mainly found in fruits and vegetables, grains, and milk and dairy foods.

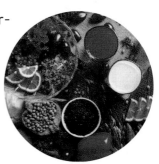

Fat-soluble vitamins—A, D, E, and K—require fat for absorption. Fat-soluble vitamins are mainly found in animal fats, vegetable oils, dairy foods, liver, and oily fish. While your body needs these vitamins to work properly, you don't need to eat foods containing them every day.

WATER-SOLUBLE VITAMINS	FAT-SOLUBLE VITAMINS
Biotin (vitamin B7)	Vitamin A
Folic acid (folate, vitamin B9)	Vitamin D
Niacin (vitamin B3)	Vitamin E
Pantothenic acid (vitamin B5)	Vitamin K
Riboflavin (vitamin B2)	
Thiamin (vitamin B1)	
Vitamin B6	
Vitamin B12	
Vitamin C	

Vitamin Deficiencies

Vitamin deficiencies have been linked to all sorts of health problems, including heart disease, anemia, osteoporosis, scurvy, rickets, and cancer. Fortunately, serious vitamin deficiencies are rare in the United States today. A 2012 nutrition report from the Centers for Disease Control and Prevention (CDC) found that overall, less than 10 percent of the U.S. population was deficient in each nutrient.

Concern about vitamin deficiencies is rapidly being replaced with concern about the effects of marginally adequate vitamin intakes—amounts that may not cause a vitamin-deficiency disease but might interfere with normal body functions.

A subclinical deficiency can sneak up on you when the amount of a nutrient in your diet or your total "body pool" of a nutrient is only marginally adequate. Biochemical and metabolic changes can begin to take place, and then you become at risk for a vitamin deficiency.

Waiting to act on your nutrient needs until you have a clear deficiency or a disease is not a prudent approach. One way to protect yourself from the dangers of undetectable subclinical deficiencies is to eat a wide variety of foods. If you do not eat enough calories, or if your eating habits are not as good as you would like, you may want to consider taking a multivitamin-mineral supplement. The supplement should balance what you are already getting from your diet. Always consult your health care provider before starting any supplements.

Vitamin Toxicity

We know that large doses of vitamins can have harmful effects on the body. In fact, an overdose of a vitamin can be as serious as a vitamin deficiency. Overdoses are more likely to occur with fat-soluble vitamins, which are stored in body fat and the liver and used as needed. The more fat-soluble vitamins you take, the more of them your body stores. If too much is stored, serious consequences result. For example, cases of toxicity from excesses of vitamins A and D are occasionally reported. (See Chapter 6 for the vitamin A and vitamin D profiles.)

Our bodies cannot store large amounts of water-soluble vitamins, so we need a more constant supply of them. Overdoses are unlikely, because we excrete any excess of these vitamins in urine if too much is consumed. Because of this, nutritionists used to believe you couldn't take in a dangerous amount of water-soluble vitamins. We now know, however, that large quantities of vitamin C and some of the B vitamins—particularly B_6—can trigger toxic effects.

Moreover, high doses of vitamins can create vitamin imbalances. That is, large amounts of one vitamin can cause a deficiency of another. For example, animal studies have shown that high doses of vitamin E may adversely affect a person's vitamin K status. Hypervitaminosis is the clinical term for a vitamin overdose. The danger of this condition exists whenever you take large doses—called megadoses—of vitamins.

So Much from So Little

Many vitamins, especially those of the B complex, act as coenzymes, or small molecules attached to enzymes that help the enzymes do their job. An enzyme is a catalyst—a substance that regulates the speed of a chemical reaction without being used up or changed in that reaction. So our bodies can use enzymes over and over again to control specific reactions. The body can also repeatedly use vitamins that act as coenzymes.

However, the body still needs a regular supply of these and the other vitamins to replace those excreted in the urine or destroyed or changed by the body during certain metabolic processes.

Vitamin-like Substances

There are other substances in food that function much like vitamins. They do not really fit the definition of vitamins, however, either because our bodies can make them or because we require them in larger amounts than we do vitamins. These substances occur so widely in foods that a deficiency is unlikely. Vitamin-like substances include choline, bioflavonoids, inositol, lipoic acid, carnitine, coenzyme Q10, and para-aminobenzoic acid (PABA). See the nutrient profiles in Chapter 6 for more on these substances.

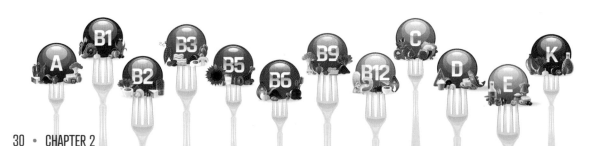

CHAPTER 3
Minerals

Minerals, also referred to as inorganic elements, make up about four percent—or about five pounds—of the body's weight. Even ancient peoples recognized the value and usefulness of minerals:

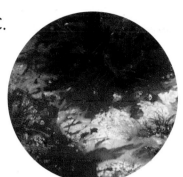

- Chinese writings from as early as 3000 B.C. recommended seaweed and burnt sponge to treat goiter, a deficiency of the mineral iodine. Seaweed and sponges are rich in iodine.

- In ancient Greece, people soaked hot iron swords in water and then used the iron-enriched water to treat anemia.

- As many as 30 references to salt—sodium chloride—can be found in the Bible, including its use in purifying ceremonies and as an offering to God.

- A Greek slave said to be "worth his weight in salt" actually commanded this price—payment in salt.

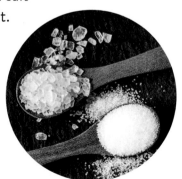

- At banquets, important people sat at the table closest to the saltcellar. This was considered a position of honor.

- The word salary is from the Latin word for salt, *saleria*.

Despite all these early references to minerals, many centuries passed before researchers clarified the role that minerals play in the body. In 1799, the French chemist Antoine-Laurent Lavoisier—often called "the father of modern chemistry"—predicted correctly that scientists would isolate "elements" from the earth.

In 1804, Swiss chemist Nicolas-Théodore de Saussure (*pictured on left*) proved that the mineral makeup of soil influenced the mineral content of plants grown in that soil. Research during the second half of the 19th century concentrated mostly on trace minerals—those needed only in tiny amounts. In the early 20th century, as scientists isolated and identified vitamins, they also demonstrated that many minerals were essential to better health and nutrition.

Today, we are aware of about 50 minerals in the body. Of these, 17 are considered essential. The others are accidental contaminants or are waiting for us to discover their true importance. Recently, for example, researchers linked boron to mineral metabolism and bone development. Even small amounts of arsenic may prove useful to the body; its role has been linked to the metabolism of the amino acid methionine.

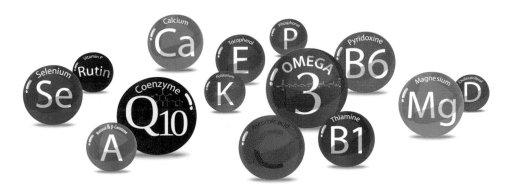

What Are Minerals?

Minerals are different from vitamins; they are not organic substances made by plants or animals. They're actually inorganic elements found in soil. Plants absorb minerals directly from the soil, and animals get their supply indirectly, either by eating the plants or by eating other animals that have eaten the plants.

There are two kinds of minerals—macrominerals and trace minerals. Minerals are grouped into these two categories depending on the amount found in the body. You need larger amounts of macrominerals (also called major minerals). They include calcium, phosphorus, magnesium, sodium, potassium, chloride, and sulfur. You only need small amounts of trace minerals (also called microminerals). They include iron, manganese, copper, iodine, zinc, cobalt, fluoride, and selenium.

For many trace minerals, there is a fine line between not enough and too much. Most of the benefits attributed to minerals come from consuming the normal amounts found in foods. Unless you are correcting a deficiency under a doctor's supervision, taking more than the recommended amount of a mineral may do more harm than good.

MACROMINERALS
Calcium
Chloride
Magnesium
Phosphorus
Potassium
Sodium
Sulfur

TRACE MINERALS
Chromium
Cobalt
Copper
Fluoride
Iodine
Iron
Manganese
Molybdenum
Selenium
Zinc

What Minerals Do

Did you know that every cell in the body contains minerals? In fact, almost everything the body does involves minerals in some way or another. Their main functions are to help maintain the structure of living tissue and to regulate important body processes.

In their structural role, minerals contribute strength and firmness to bones and teeth. They're also part of essential body compounds. For example, iron is a part of hemoglobin (the oxygen-carrying substance in red blood cells) and is also a part of a number of different enzymes; iodine is a part of the thyroid hormone; and cobalt is a part of vitamin B$_{12}$.

In their role as regulators, minerals act as cofactors in enzyme-controlled body reactions. In other words, they keep enzyme reactions running up to speed. Iron, zinc, and copper are parts of enzymes. If the diet doesn't supply enough of these minerals, the body can't make enough enzymes.

Free mineral ions—particles with either a positive or negative electrical charge—have many important functions. These ions are important for maintenance of normal acid-base balance, transmission of nerve impulses, regulation of normal cell membrane function, and regulation of muscle response to nerve stimuli.

Some minerals have drug-like effects. For example, fluoride prevents tooth decay and chromium can help control blood sugar in people with diabetes.

Mineral Deficiencies

Nutrition surveys occasionally find that intake of certain minerals, such as calcium, potassium, iron, and zinc, are lower than recommended. A mineral deficiency often happens slowly over time. Common causes of deficiencies include an increased need for the mineral, lack of the mineral in the diet, or difficulty absorbing the mineral from food.

Many food manufacturers replace some of the minerals lost during processing. This process is called enrichment. In the 1920s, health authorities successfully prevented iodine-deficiency goiter by adding iodine to salt. Manufacturers frequently add iron to cereals and breads that have the mineral stripped during processing. Many companies add calcium to fruit juices, breakfast cereals, and breads, too. The best way to prevent or remedy nutrient deficiencies is to make sure you're eating a balanced, nutrient-rich diet.

Mineral Toxicity

Mineral toxicity is a condition where the concentration of a mineral in the body is abnormally high, and where there is an adverse effect on health. Excessive mineral supplements can be harmful. Large doses can cause abnormal fluid accumulations in vital organs, interfere with the functions of other minerals, and irritate the intestines, which may cause nausea and bleeding. A real danger is the replacement of one mineral with a similar one in an enzyme. The impostor enzyme doesn't function as the real one does, or it doesn't function at all.

A Word About Water

In the body, metabolic reactions involving vitamins and minerals take place in water. Thus, water is essential for the maintenance of normal body function. Water makes up about 60 percent of an adult's body and an even greater percentage of a child's body. Men have slightly more water in their bodies than women do, and younger people have more than older people. About 70 percent of lean body tissue, or muscle, is actually water.

Water carries nutrients into cells and transports wastes out of them. It acts as a solvent for compounds such as vitamins, minerals, glucose, and amino acids (the building blocks of protein). It lubricates joints, acts as a shock absorber inside the eyes and spinal cord, and helps the body maintain its temperature.

Most people drink about 2½ quarts of water daily. Normally, this comes from many sources: liquids (milk, tap water, non-caffeinated soft drinks, soups), animal foods (meat, fish, eggs), and fruits and vegetables. Moisture in foods accounts for about 20 percent of total water intake. For example, cucumbers are about 96 percent water; lettuce, 94 percent; watermelon, 93 percent; broccoli, 91 percent; and oranges, 84 percent.

We lose water in urine, stool, sweat, and the air we exhale. People who are healthy generally excrete at least one quart of urine a day to rid the body of wastes. During waking hours, this means urinating about every four hours. Less frequent urination is a sign you're not consuming enough fluids.

Thirst partially controls the water content of the body, but often thirst lags behind the body's needs. That makes it even more important to pay attention to your thirst. When you thirst for water, you're usually already behind in fluid intake.

So indulge yourself (unless your doctor has advised you to do otherwise). Drinking too much water poses no danger to healthy people; they just excrete the excess, producing more dilute urine.

Electrolytes

When found in body tissues, minerals occur mainly as mineral salts. When these mineral salts dissolve in water, they may separate into ions—electrically charged particles called electrolytes. Sodium and potassium are the body's major electrolytes. They are extremely important. Electrolytes help control the flow of nutrients into and waste products out of cells.

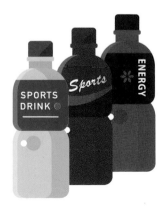

CHAPTER 4
Antioxidants

The antioxidant story begins with oxygen. We all know that oxygen is essential for life. Every cell in the body requires oxygen to get energy from nutrients. Without it, our bodies would simply shut down. Ironically, though, the very same oxygen molecules that keep us alive are easily turned into rogue particles that can leave a path of destruction throughout the body. The damage they cause sets the stage for a variety of diseases and, scientists suspect, prompts many of the changes we associate with aging.

How can something so vital become so harmful? When an oxygen molecule is in its normal, beneficial form, the electrons in its chemical structure are paired off. If that oxygen molecule loses one of its electrons, however, it becomes unstable—and destructive. This unstable molecule is called a *free radical*.

A free radical wants nothing more than to replace its missing electron, and it will steal one from wherever it can. If it robs a nearby oxygen molecule, that molecule becomes an unstable free radical. That destabilized molecule may, in turn, grab an electron from another molecule, causing a free-radical chain reaction. Alternately, an oxygen free radical may attack a nearby healthy cell, punching a hole in the cell's membrane to steal an electron and causing damage that may remain, even if the assaulted cell is able to replace its missing electron. The process in which oxygen free radicals assault stable molecules or healthy cells is called *oxidation*.

Free radicals can damage any tissue or organ, as well as any fat, protein, or carbohydrate molecule, in the body. The "victims" may include DNA, the genetic material that regulates cell growth; the fat molecules in every cell's protective membrane; the low-density lipoprotein (LDL) molecules that carry cholesterol in the bloodstream; and the proteins that help form the structure of the heart, blood vessels, muscles, skin, and other tissue. Down the road, these kinds of insults may accumulate and lead to inflammation, abnormal or uncontrolled cell growth, hardening of the arteries, and other disease-inducing changes. Among the diseases thought to be associated with free-radical damage are cancer, cardiovascular diseases, diabetes, Parkinson's disease, cataracts and age-related macular degeneration, and Alzheimer's disease and certain other dementias.

HELP ME—I'M RUSTING!

The oxidation process is not unique to humans. In fact, it is the human equivalent of rusting. Metals form rust when their ordinarily stable molecules are oxidized. Other examples of oxidation include the browning of fruit when the flesh contacts air and the spoiling (rancidity) of cooking oils that eventually occurs once the airtight seals on their bottles have been opened.

How does an oxygen molecule lose an electron in the first place? Sometimes, the loss occurs during the body's normal use of oxygen for metabolic processes. In other words, some free radicals are simply natural byproducts of living. But far more often, exposure to environmental toxins such as air pollution, cigarette smoke, and the sun's ultraviolet (UV) rays results in the creation of free radicals.

Fortunately, our bodies have a natural defense mechanism against free-radical damage. The key element of that mechanism is a class of molecular compounds called antioxidants. Antioxidants neutralize free radicals, either by shielding healthy cells or by halting free-radical chain reactions. We have a number of antioxidant defenders at our disposal, each with its own protective functions. Some come in the form of vitamins and minerals. Vitamin C, vitamin E, and beta-carotene (a form of vitamin A) are antioxidants, as are the minerals selenium, manganese, and zinc. In addition, special chemicals from plants, called *phytochemicals*, can act as antioxidants in our bodies. We arm ourselves with these natural protective chemicals by eating a diet rich in plant foods, including vegetables, fruits, whole grains, legumes, and nuts.

Unfortunately, this antioxidant defense mechanism is not foolproof. It typically has little difficulty keeping up with the free radicals created by normal bodily functions, but it can be overwhelmed when we expose ourselves to too many environmental toxins and/or don't replenish our antioxidant stores by regularly consuming enough minimally processed plant foods (processing, as well as overcooking, tends to strip plant foods of some of their natural antioxidants). The resulting oxidative stress is thought to set the stage for the various diseases associated with free-radical damage. The good news is we can reduce our exposure to many environmental causes of free radicals. Plus, we can bolster our defenses against free-radical damage by boosting our dietary intake of antioxidants.

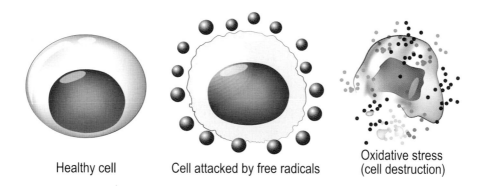

Healthy cell   Cell attacked by free radicals   Oxidative stress
                                                               (cell destruction)

How Do Antioxidants Work?

Antioxidants tackle free radicals by using a variety of tactics. One strategy is to run interference between the free radical and the cell material it has targeted to attack for an electron. By giving the free radical one of its own electrons, the antioxidant spares the cell material from damage. Antioxidants that work this way are called free-radical scavengers. Vitamin C, beta-carotene, and vitamin E all work as scavengers.

Mineral antioxidants use another tactic. These minerals are attached to cell proteins called enzymes. The enzymes take out the free radicals through chemical reactions. Selenium works with an enzyme called glutathione peroxidase, while zinc works with superoxide dismutase, or SOD. A protein in the blood called ceruloplasmin, which contains copper, may also act as an antioxidant. Each of these enzymes has a particular free radical it keeps under surveillance.

The various antioxidants cooperate with one another to achieve their goal of protection against free-radical damage. They require this team effort because antioxidants exist in different places in the cell and attack different free radicals. Vitamin E usually protects the fat in the cell membranes, while vitamin C protects mostly proteins. Beta-carotene is the most powerful defense we have against free radicals formed by ultraviolet light. Selenium enzymes protect the cell machinery that generates energy. Zinc enzymes take up stations at other points to halt free radicals that might have slipped by other antioxidants.

Vitamin C also helps put vitamin E back in action by giving it another electron once vitamin E loses its electron to a free radical. Likewise, vitamin E steps in to help out if selenium supplies are insufficient. So taking in enough selenium frees vitamin E to be more effective in its other duties.

Are We Getting Enough?

Even if you eat food sources of antioxidants, it does not always guarantee that your body will get sufficient amounts. Citrus fruits, strawberries, potatoes, green peppers, and tomatoes contain substantial amounts of vitamin C, but high temperatures destroy the vitamin when these foods are heated.

Yellow-orange fruits and vegetables, such as carrots, squash, apricots, and mangoes, are concentrated sources of beta-carotene. Dark-green, leafy vegetables such as spinach, broccoli, asparagus, and mustard or beet greens are also rich in beta-carotene. High temperatures do not destroy this compound, and cooking may, in fact, make beta-carotene in plant foods more available. Extended storage in sunlight or exposure to the air, however, can destroy beta-carotene.

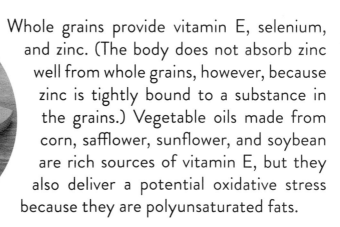

Whole grains provide vitamin E, selenium, and zinc. (The body does not absorb zinc well from whole grains, however, because zinc is tightly bound to a substance in the grains.) Vegetable oils made from corn, safflower, sunflower, and soybean are rich sources of vitamin E, but they also deliver a potential oxidative stress because they are polyunsaturated fats.

Supplement Pitfalls

Research has found that people who eat more antioxidant-rich vegetables and fruits have lower risks of several diseases. Many assumed that because these foods are rich in antioxidants, then antioxidants must be the protective factor. However, it's not clear whether the results are related to the amount of antioxidants in vegetables and fruits, to other components of these foods, to other factors in people's diets, or to other lifestyle choices.

Fruits and vegetables are also rich in fiber and low in fat. They also sport phytochemicals. It could be any one of these—or all of them together—that helps prevent disease. If you take an antioxidant supplement on the assumption that it holds the key, you eliminate the possible benefits these other substances might contribute. Besides, antioxidants work as a team to protect the body from free-radical damage. Taking extra amounts of one will not substitute for the lack of another.

Research has thus far not shown that antioxidant supplements provide the same benefits as antioxidant-rich foods in preventing diseases. Rigorous scientific studies involving large numbers of people have tested whether antioxidant supplements can help prevent chronic diseases such as cancer, cardiovascular diseases, and cataracts. In most instances, antioxidant supplements did not reduce the risks of developing these diseases.

High-dose supplements of antioxidants may be linked to health risks in some cases. For example, high doses of beta-carotene may increase the risk of lung cancer in smokers. High doses of vitamin E may increase the risks of prostate cancer and a type of stroke. Antioxidant supplements may also interact with some medicines. For example, vitamin E supplements may increase the risk of bleeding in people who are taking blood thinners.

For now it seems best to stick with food sources of antioxidants. Just be sure to eat lots of fruits and vegetables—you can't overdose on them. And one thing you'll be sure of getting is plenty of phytochemicals.

Phytochemicals to the Rescue

Phytochemicals are natural substances found in plants. *Phyto* means plant. They are neither vitamins nor minerals, but they may hold the key to optimal health. Genistein in soy foods, polyphenols in tea, psoralens in celery, sulforaphane in broccoli, allylic sulfides in garlic, and ellagic acid in strawberries—these are just a few of the exciting discoveries.

Scientists are busy trying to identify these and other phytochemicals and to discover just what they do. The task is daunting. An orange alone contains some 150 phytochemicals that provide various benefits.

To benefit from phytochemicals, you need only to start eating more fruits and vegetables. You've probably heard the call to eat five servings per day. That's just the beginning. The real goal, experts say, is to eat five to nine servings of fruits and vegetables a day. Until now, researchers have focused on the beta-carotene and fiber in fruits and vegetables as the reason for their protective effect, but maybe that's not all there is to it. Maybe they have something else in common. Enter phytochemicals.

Carotenoids, other than beta-carotene, have begun to receive more attention. A lot of the same foods rich in beta-carotene are rich in other carotenoids that appear to have anticancer effects as well. Lycopene is one of the most promising. An Italian study suggests that people who eat a lot of tomatoes may have less risk of cancers of the gastrointestinal tract. Tomatoes are rich in lycopene.

Of course, tomatoes are rich in vitamin C, too. So what is "the good stuff"? Maybe fiber is part of the equation. Or maybe the protective effect works only when these substances are all combined in the exact way they are in tomatoes. Perhaps the idea of extracting out "the good stuff " is naive. You can be assured of obtaining the best possible array of nutrients by eating the widest variety of whole fruits and vegetables you can. A winning strategy is to get "the good stuff" from eating more fruits and vegetables.

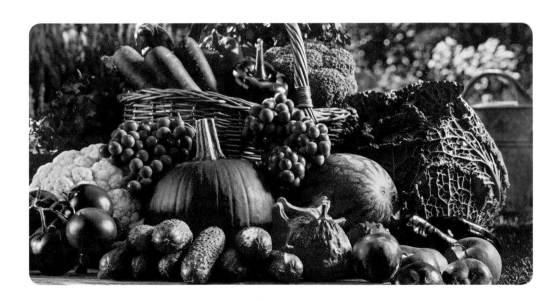

Food Sources of Antioxidants

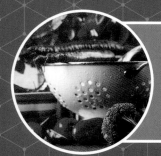

Beta-carotene
Found in sweet potatoes, carrots, winter squash, cantaloupe, apricots, sweet peppers, spinach, collard greens, kale, and broccoli.

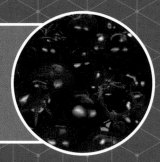

Lycopene
Especially abundant in tomatoes; also found in pink grapefruit, watermelon, red cabbage, papaya, guavas, red peppers, and apricots.

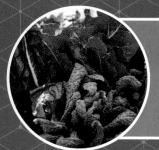

Lutein
Found in collard greens, kale, spinach, broccoli, Brussels sprouts, asparagus, green peas, papaya, corn, artichokes, and oranges.

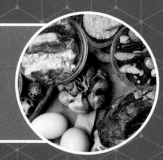

Selenium
Found in Brazil nuts, seafood, liver, meat, poultry, fish, eggs, dairy products, breads, cereals, and other grain products.

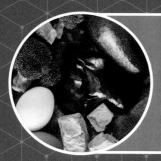

VITAMIN A
Found in sweet potatoes, liver, spinach, carrots, cantaloupe, mangoes, dairy products, broccoli, squash, pumpkin, apricots, eggs, and fortified breakfast cereals.

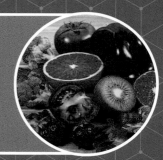

VITAMIN C
Found in citrus fruits, red and green peppers, strawberries, kiwifruit, Brussels sprouts, broccoli, cauliflower, tomatoes, tomato juice, potatoes, cantaloupe, and cabbage.

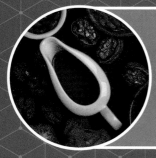

VITAMIN E
Found in vegetable oils (such as wheat germ, sunflower, and safflower oils), nuts (such as almonds, peanuts, and hazelnuts), sunflower seeds, broccoli, and fortified foods.

CHAPTER 5
Supplements

A growing number of adults in the United States take dietary supplements. Dietary supplements include vitamins and minerals, herbs and botanicals, and many other products. Supplements come in the form of pills, capsules, powders, drinks, and energy bars. Some dietary supplements may be beneficial to health. However, taking supplements may also involve health risks. Just because a product is advertised as "natural" doesn't mean it's safe.

A common perception is that because vitamins, herbs, and other supplements are natural, they are automatically gentler and don't cause side effects like drugs do. That's not always the case, however. Some do have a mild effect and don't appear to cause adverse reactions. But supplements are not as strictly regulated in the United States as are medications, so it's difficult to be sure that you're getting the ingredients and doses that you pay for. In addition, dietary supplements may cause dangerous side effects, especially if taken at high doses, taken for longer than recommended, or taken with other supplements or medicines.

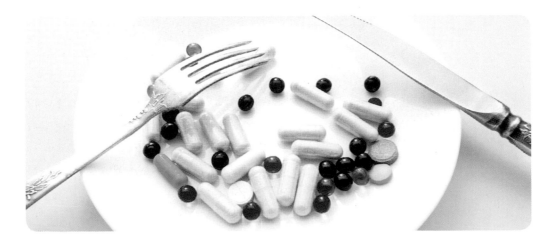

How Supplements Are Regulated

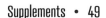

The U.S. Food and Drug Administration (FDA) regulates dietary supplements differently than prescription and over-the-counter drugs. Before marketing a drug, manufacturers must obtain FDA approval by providing convincing evidence that the drug is both safe and effective. Dietary supplements are not required to be tested for safety and effectiveness before they are marketed. Dietary supplement manufacturers are required to ensure their products are produced in a quality manner, are free of contaminants and impurities, and are accurately labeled.

Once a dietary supplement is on the market, the FDA monitors information on the product's label and package insert. The Federal Trade Commission (FTC), which regulates product advertising, also requires that all information about a dietary supplement be truthful and not misleading.

Benefits

Scientific evidence shows that some dietary supplements are beneficial for health. For example, calcium and vitamin D are important for keeping bones strong. Folic acid decreases the risk of certain birth defects. Other supplements need more study.

Here are some of the groups who may benefit from supplements:

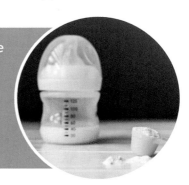

Infants need a source of iron when they reach the age of six months. Breast milk provides very little, and by this time, their body stores are depleted. Fortified cereal or formula fills the bill. A fluoride supplement is also recommended to prevent dental decay.

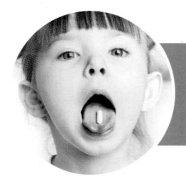

Children usually get what they need from their diet. If their eating habits tend toward long jags or if they are vegetarians, a multivitamin-mineral supplement can provide insurance.

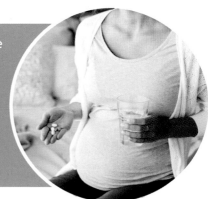

Pregnant women and women planning to conceive are good candidates for a multivitamin-mineral supplement. It's wise to be sure your nutrient levels are optimal before becoming pregnant. It's also important to meet your body's increased need for the vitamins B_6, C, and D, and the minerals calcium, copper, iron, and zinc.

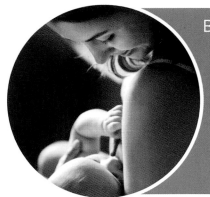

Breastfeeding women are also candidates. Although their increased nutrient requirements can largely be met by the extra food needed to meet their increased calorie needs, a supplement can help insure against depletion of the vitamins B_6, C, and D, and the minerals calcium, magnesium, and zinc. Calcium needs may dictate a separate supplement.

Vegans and children who are vegetarians may not get all the nutrients their bodies need. Most vegetarians are no more likely to need a supplement than anyone else, but the exceptions may be growing children and adult vegans (who also shun dairy and eggs in addition to meat, fish, and poultry). They may need other sources of vitamin B_{12}, vitamin D, calcium, iron, and zinc.

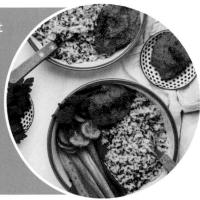

Seniors older than 50 years of age need more of some nutrients and less of others, so they shouldn't pop pills indiscriminately. They need more folate and vitamins B_6, B_{12}, and D, though the body may have its own mechanisms for filling the B_{12} and folate gaps. Some also think it's wise for seniors to up their intake of the antioxidant vitamins C and E and beta-carotene. Postmenopausal women almost certainly need a calcium supplement. Based on the latest Dietary Reference Intake recommendations, women in this group should get 1,200 milligrams per day.

Risks

Dietary supplements are not intended to treat, diagnose, mitigate, prevent, or cure disease. In some cases, dietary supplements may have unwanted effects. Supplements are most likely to cause side effects when taken instead of prescribed medicines or in combination with many other supplements.

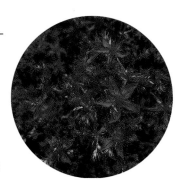

ST. JOHN'S WORT

- Some dietary supplements interact with medications (prescription or over-the-counter). For example, St. John's wort makes many medications less effective.

- Antioxidant supplements, like vitamins C and E, might reduce the effectiveness of some types of cancer chemotherapy.

- Certain dietary supplements may increase the risk of bleeding or affect a person's response to anesthesia when taken before or after surgery.

- Pregnant or nursing women and children should be cautious about taking dietary supplements. Most dietary supplements have not been tested in pregnant women, nursing mothers, or children.

- More isn't always better. Taking too much of some vitamins and minerals can cause health problems. For example, taking too much vitamin A can cause birth defects, reduce bone strength, and lead to liver damage.

- Product contamination is a serious risk. Hundreds of supplements have been found to contain hidden drugs and other chemicals, particularly in products for weight loss, sexual health, and bodybuilding.

- "Natural" doesn't always mean "safe." For example, the herbs comfrey and kava can harm the liver.

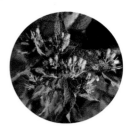

COMFREY

- What's on the label may not be what's in the bottle. Analyses of dietary supplements have found differences between labeled and actual ingredients.

- Don't take supplements in place of, or in combination with, prescribed medications without consulting your health care provider.

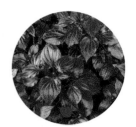

KAVA

Checking the Label

All products labeled as dietary supplements have a Supplement Facts panel that lists the serving size, dietary ingredients, amount per serving, and Percent of Daily Value (%DV), if established. Non-dietary ingredients, such as fillers, artificial colors, sweeteners, flavors, or binders, are also listed on the label. The amounts of the nutrients in a supplement are given in milligrams (mg), micrograms (mcg or µg), or international units (IU).

Dietary supplement labels can make some health-related claims. Manufacturers are allowed to say, for example, that a dietary supplement addresses a nutrient deficiency, supports health, or is linked to a particular body function. But such claims must be followed by "This statement has not been evaluated by the Food and Drug Administration. This product is not intended to diagnose, treat, cure, or prevent any disease."

Foods vs. Supplements

Wouldn't it be nice to meet all your nutritional needs by swallowing a single pill? Unfortunately, it doesn't work that way. Supplements, by definition, are there to supplement a diet, not substitute for it. Food is essential to good health. Although we know something about food and the components that are vital to good health, we 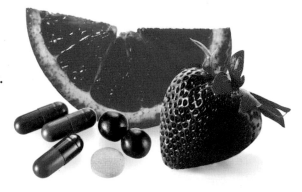 will never know everything. For example, scientists have already identified more than 10,000 non-nutrient compounds in plant foods. These compounds may not be essential, but each has shown some positive effects on health.

Food is also preferable to supplements as a primary source of vitamins and minerals because it's much more difficult to get too much of a vitamin or a mineral from food, making overdosing unlikely. At the very high doses typical of megadose supplements, the drug-like effects of nutrients can be harmful. Although toxicity rarely causes death, it can cause considerable discomfort and interfere with the healthy functioning of the body.

Aim to get your intake of vitamins and minerals from food rather than a pill. Eating a wide variety of foods is the best way to meet your nutrient needs. Talk with your health care provider before taking any supplements.

CHAPTER 6
Nutrient Profiles

AMINO ACIDS

Amino acids are the building blocks of protein. Together they form the proteins in foods that enable our bodies to grow and maintain tissues, antibodies, hormones, blood cells, and neurotransmitters—the chemical messengers that allow the nerves to send signals throughout the body. Neurotransmitters are especially concentrated in the brain. Therapeutic use of amino acids often focuses on their ability to influence the production of these powerful chemicals.

There are two kinds of amino acids: essential and nonessential. Essential amino acids cannot be made by the body and so must be obtained through the diet. Nonessential amino acids can be made in sufficient amounts by the body and therefore are not required in the diet.

Supplementation can be tricky because large amounts of one amino acid often prevent another amino acid from doing its job. An imbalance can have undesired health consequences. For that reason, a health care provider who can monitor levels of the amino acids and keep them in balance should supervise amino acid supplementation.

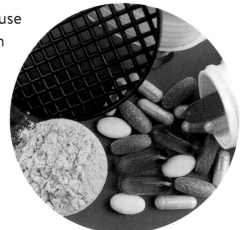

ANTIOXIDANTS

As discussed in Chapter 4, antioxidants are substances that help protect cells from damage caused by free radicals. Free radicals are naturally formed when you exercise and when your body converts food into energy. You can also be exposed to free radicals from environmental sources, such as tobacco smoke, sunlight, and pollution. Antioxidants include vitamins A, C, and E, beta-carotene, lutein, lycopene, selenium, and zinc. See Chapter 4 for more about antioxidants.

B VITAMINS

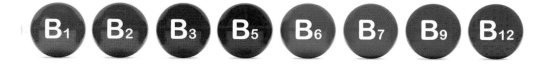

B vitamins are a group of water-soluble vitamins that are important for cell function. The B vitamins are: thiamin (vitamin B_1), riboflavin (vitamin B_2), niacin (vitamin B_3), pantothenic acid (vitamin B_5), vitamin B_6, biotin (vitamin B_7), folate (vitamin B_9), and vitamin B_{12}. These eight vitamins make up the vitamin B complex. B vitamins are found in yeast, seeds, eggs, liver, meat, and vegetables.

BETA-CAROTENE (VITAMIN A)

Beta-carotene is one of a group of red, orange, and yellow pigments called carotenoids. The body converts beta-carotene into vitamin A, an essential nutrient needed for healthy eyes and skin, normal growth and development, and immune system function. Like all carotenoids, beta-carotene is an antioxidant. Antioxidants help fight against free radicals.

Sources of Beta-Carotene

Beta-carotene is found in orange, red, and yellow plant foods and in some dark green vegetables. Good sources of beta-carotene include carrots, sweet potatoes, pumpkin, collard greens, spinach, kale, broccoli, winter squash, cantaloupe, and apricots.

Beta-carotene is included in some anti-oxidant and multivitamin supplements, and is also available in separate beta-carotene supplements. Beta-carotene supplements are not recommended for general use. Don't take beta-carotene supplements if you smoke.

Beta-Carotene and Health

Beta-carotene can reduce sun sensitivity in people with erythropoietic protoporphyria, an inherited blood disorder. Beta-carotene may also help prevent age-related macular degeneration, breast cancer, pregnancy-related complications, and sunburn.

While people who eat a lot of foods containing beta-carotene might have a lower risk of certain kinds of cancer, studies have not yet shown that vitamin A or beta-carotene supplements can help prevent cancer.

BILBERRY

Bilberry is a deciduous shrub with thin, creeping stems. Leaves are bright green, alternate, and oval. Flowers are pale green to pink and appear from late spring to late summer, followed by purple fruit. Native to Europe, northern Asia, and North America, the herb is found in woodlands, forests, and moorlands. One of more than 100 members of the genus *Vaccinium*, bilberry is related to blueberries and huckleberries.

Bilberry contains vitamins A and C and was a folk remedy in Scandinavia to prevent scurvy and treat nausea and indigestion. The berries were once steeped in gin and taken as a digestive tonic. They are a popular Russian remedy for colitis and stomach ulcers because they decrease inflammation in the intestines and protect the lining of the digestive tract. The herb has astringent, antiseptic, and tonic properties, making it useful as a treatment for diarrhea.

Berries contain flavonoid anthocyanidins, which have a potent antioxidant action and protect body tissues, particularly blood vessels. Several studies have shown that bilberry extracts stimulate blood vessels to release a substance that helps dilate (open) veins and arteries. Bilberries may keep platelets from clumping, thus preventing clotting and improving circulation. The berry may help prevent many diabetes-related conditions caused by poor circulation.

Because they contain a substance that slightly lowers blood sugar, the leaves are a folk remedy to manage diabetes. However, you should not use the leaves to self-treat diabetes. German researchers are investigating the leaves as a treatment for gout and rheumatism.

Bilberry preparations may be particularly useful for treating eye conditions and have been prescribed for diabetic retinopathy, cataracts, night blindness, and macular degeneration. In England, World War II pilots were given bilberry jam to improve their eyesight. Modern European prescription medications that contain bilberry are used to improve eyesight and circulation.

Today, bilberry dietary supplements are used for cardiovascular conditions, diarrhea, urinary tract infections, eye problems, and diabetes, among other conditions. You can buy bilberry extract in tablets, capsules, and drops. The berries are dried and sold as a powder. The leaves are made into teas. While the fruit (when consumed in amounts typically found in foods) and the extract (in recommended doses for brief periods of time) are generally considered safe, bilberry leaves taken orally in high doses or for long periods of time may be unsafe.

BIOFLAVONOIDS

Citrus fruits and their skins are the secret hiding places of bioflavonoids. In the 1930s, nutritionists believed bioflavonoids could reverse the effects of vitamin C deficiency. This idea was later proved wrong; there is no evidence that bioflavonoids are essential to normal functioning. They may, however, prove to have some disease-preventing powers.

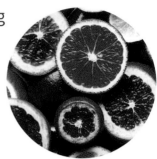

BIOTIN (VITAMIN B7)

Biotin is a B vitamin found in many foods, including eggs, meats, and milk. Biotin helps convert the carbohydrates, fats, and proteins in food into energy.

History

In the 1930s, an investigator at the Lister Institute of Preventive Medicine in London, England, was experimenting with the diets of rats. After feeding the rodents raw egg whites for several weeks, he noticed they developed an eczema-like skin condition, lost their hair, became paralyzed, and began to hemorrhage under the skin.

Later, another team of investigators fed rats different foods to see which ones prevented or alleviated the "egg-white syndrome." Various foods, such as dried yeast, milk, and egg yolk, were successful in curing the rats' conditions. But what did all of these foods have in common?

It was 1940 before scientist Paul Gyorgy identified the common denominator as a vitamin. At first, thinking that it was an isolated substance, he named it vitamin H. Soon after, however, scientists realized it was actually another member of the B complex family. They soon did away with vitamin H and renamed the vitamin biotin (or vitamin B_7).

Functions of Biotin

Biotin acts as a coenzyme in several metabolic reactions. It plays a role in the manufacture of body fats, the metabolism of carbohydrates, the breakdown of proteins to urea, and the conversion of amino acids from protein into blood sugar for energy.

Sources of Biotin

Milk, liver, eggs, seeds, meats, and fish are sources of biotin. Nuts and mushrooms contain smaller amounts of the vitamin. Bacteria in the intestine also make biotin.

FOOD SOURCES OF BIOTIN

FOOD	QUANTITY	MICROGRAMS
Beef liver, raw	3½ ounces	100 mcg
Cauliflower	1 cup	17 mcg
Egg, cooked	1 whole	10 mcg
Blue cheese	3½ ounces	7 mcg
Skim milk (nonfat)	1 cup	5 mcg
Sardines, in oil	3½ ounces	5 mcg
Banana	1 medium	4 mcg
Grapefruit	½ medium	3 mcg

Recommended Intakes for Biotin

Recommended intakes for biotin and other nutrients come from the Dietary Reference Intakes, which are developed by the Food and Nutrition Board at the National Academies of Sciences, Engineering, and Medicine. The Adequate Intake (AI) levels for biotin are shown in the table below. (Adequate Intakes are established when evidence is insufficient to develop a Recommended Dietary Allowance, or RDA.)

ADEQUATE INTAKES (AIs) FOR BIOTIN

LIFE STAGE GROUP	MICROGRAMS PER DAY
Infants 0–6 months	5 mcg
Infants 7–12 months	6 mcg
Children 1–3 years	8 mcg
Children 4–8 years	12 mcg
Children 9–13 years	20 mcg
Teens 14–18 years	25 mcg
Adults 19+ years	30 mcg
Pregnant teens and women	30 mcg
Breastfeeding teens and women	35 mcg

Deficiency of Biotin

A true biotin deficiency is rare in the United States. However, certain groups of people are more likely to have an inadequate intake of biotin, including people with a rare genetic disorder called biotinidase deficiency, people with alcohol dependence, and women who are pregnant or breastfeeding.

Biotin Use and Misuse

Biotin supplements may be needed in rare instances. Recently, however, it has been touted as a vitamin that can improve the health of your hair, skin, and nails. But there is little scientific evidence to back up these claims.

Large intakes of biotin have not been found to be toxic. However, supplementing with biotin beyond recommended intakes can cause false results in some laboratory tests.

Biotin can interact with certain medications, and some medications may affect biotin levels. For example, treatment for at least one year with anticonvulsant (antiseizure) medications can significantly lower biotin levels.

BORON

Boron is a trace mineral found in food and in the environment. Boron appears to affect the way the body handles other minerals such as magnesium, calcium, and phosphorus. It also appears to increase estrogen levels in postmenopausal women and healthy men. Boric acid, which is a common form of boron, can kill yeast that cause vaginal infections. Some people take boron supplements for painful periods. No Recommended Dietary Allowance (RDA) for boron exists because no clear biological function has been found.

CALCIUM

Functions of Calcium

Building strong bones and teeth is the most familiar function of calcium. Indeed, those bones and teeth contain 99 percent of all the calcium in your body. The remaining one percent circulates in blood or resides in the body's soft tissues. This one percent, however, plays many extremely important roles. It participates in blood clotting, contraction and relaxation of muscles, transmission of nerve impulses, activation of enzymes, and hormone secretion.

Because maintaining a normal blood calcium level is so important to vital functions such as heart rhythm, the body has a way to ensure a constant level of calcium in the blood, no matter how much your diet provides. The secret reservoir of calcium happens to be your bones, which release calcium into the blood as needed. But if this happens too rapidly, your bones suffer the consequences.

Sources of Calcium

Milk, yogurt, cheese, and other dairy products are rich sources of calcium. Dried beans and peas and green vegetables such as broccoli, kale, bok choy, and chard are also good sources.

Phytic acid, a substance found in whole grains, can reduce calcium absorption. Oxalic acid, which is found in some vegetables and beans, can also reduce calcium absorption. Vitamin D increases calcium absorption.

Many fruit juices and drinks, cereals, and tofu are now fortified with calcium. Fruit juices contain acids, such as citric acid, that boost the amount of calcium absorbed. For someone who does not, or cannot, drink milk, orange juice fortified with calcium can be a nutritious alternative.

The USDA's MyPlate food guidance system recommends that people eat 3 cups of foods from the dairy group per day. A cup is equal to 1 cup (8 ounces) of milk, 1 cup of yogurt, 1.5 ounces of natural cheese (such as Cheddar), or 2 ounces of processed cheese (such as American).

FOOD SOURCES OF CALCIUM

FOOD	QUANTITY	MILLIGRAMS
Plain yogurt, low-fat	8 ounces	415 mg
Mozzarella, part skim	1.5 ounces	333 mg
Cheddar cheese	1.5 ounces	307 mg
Soymilk, calcium fortified	1 cup	299 mg
Skim milk (nonfat)	1 cup	299 mg
Reduced-fat milk (2%)	1 cup	293 mg
Orange juice, calcium fortified	6 ounces	261 mg
Tofu, firm, made with calcium sulfate	½ cup	253 mg
Turnip greens, fresh, boiled	½ cup	99 mg

Recommended Intakes for Calcium

The Recommended Dietary Allowance (RDA) for adults ranges from 1,000 to 1,300 milligrams (mg) of calcium daily. For women ages 19–50 who are pregnant or breastfeeding, the RDA is 1,000 mg. This is also the requirement for children ages 4–8, adults ages 19–50, and men ages 51–70.

No RDA has been established for infants. The established Adequate Intake (AI) for infants from birth to 6 months of age is 200 mg per day; 260 mg per day is the AI for infants 7–12 months old.

Certain groups are more likely to have an inadequate intake of calcium. Groups that don't get recommended amounts of calcium from foods include boys ages 9–13, girls ages 9–18, women over 50 years old, and men over 70 years old. Even when considering total calcium intakes from both food and supplements, many adolescent girls still fall short of getting enough calcium. Some older women, on the other hand, likely exceed the upper limit when both food and supplements are included.

RECOMMENDED DIETARY ALLOWANCES (RDAs) FOR CALCIUM

LIFE STAGE GROUP	MILLIGRAMS PER DAY
Infants 0–6 months	200 mg*
Infants 7–12 months	260 mg*
Children 1–3 years	700 mg
Children 4–8 years	1,000 mg
Children and teens 9–18 years	1,300 mg
Adults 19–50 years	1,000 mg
Men 51–70 years	1,000 mg
Women 51–70 years	1,200 mg
Adults 71+ years	1,200 mg
Pregnant and breastfeeding teens 14–18 years	1,300 mg
Pregnant and breastfeeding women 19–50 years	1,000 mg

*Adequate Intake (AI)

Deficiency of Calcium

A deficiency of calcium can stunt the development of bones and teeth. A lack of vitamin D, which is needed for calcium's absorption and use, can have a similar effect. Without it, there's a softening of bones, called rickets in children and osteomalacia in adults.

Bones suffer the brunt of insufficient calcium because they defer their needs to other functions that demand a higher priority. Blood clotting and muscle contraction are critical functions of calcium that must be sustained to preserve life. If muscle contractions go awry, your heart can stop. So when the blood contains too little calcium, bones give up their calcium for these functions. If this happens too often, bones become porous and weak.

The result of such weakening is osteoporosis. Osteoporosis is a condition in which bones become porous, fragile, and prone to fracture. Of the estimated 10 million Americans ages 50 and over with osteoporosis, about 80 percent are women. In men, the condition is less common because they have a larger bone mass to work with and generally take in more calcium. Low calcium and vitamin D intakes during childhood, teen, and early adult years can set the stage for osteoporosis in later life.

Calcium Use and Misuse

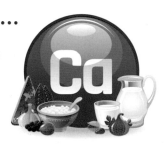

Doctors correct a calcium deficiency with calcium supplements, which often have vitamin D added to ensure calcium absorption. Doctors also prescribe calcium supplements to postmenopausal women to prevent osteoporosis, since it can be difficult to get the recommended amount of calcium.

Some studies have found that getting recommended intakes of calcium can reduce the risk of developing high blood pressure. Taking calcium supplements during pregnancy may reduce the risk of preeclampsia.

High calcium intake can cause constipation. It may also interfere with the body's ability to absorb iron and zinc, though the link is not well established. Calcium supplements can interact or interfere with several types of medications, and some medications can lower or raise calcium levels in the body. Talk to your health care providers about any supplements and medications you take.

CARNITINE

Carnitine is the general name for a number of compounds that include L-carnitine, acetyl-L-carnitine, and propionyl-L-carnitine. Carnitine plays a role in fat and energy metabolism in the body.

Carnitine is found mostly in foods of animal origin; therefore, a vegetarian diet is apt to be low in carnitine. The body makes enough carnitine to meet the needs of most people. Some individuals, such as preterm babies, cannot make sufficient amounts of carnitine.

Sources of Carnitine

The best sources of carnitine are animal products like meat, fish, poultry, and milk. L-carnitine, acetyl-L-carnitine, and propionyl-L-carnitine are sold as over-the-counter dietary supplements. The U.S. Food and Drug Administration (FDA) approved carnitine as a drug to treat certain carnitine deficiencies.

Recommended Intakes for Carnitine

The Food and Nutrition Board has not established a Recommended Dietary Allowance (RDA) for carnitine. Healthy people don't need to consume any carnitine from food or supplements, as the liver and kidneys produce sufficient amounts to meet daily needs.

Deficiencies of Carnitine

There are two types of carnitine deficiency—primary and secondary. Primary carnitine deficiency is a genetic disorder that usually manifests itself by the age of 5. Secondary carnitine deficiencies may occur due to certain disorders (such as chronic renal failure) or under specific conditions (such as use of certain antibiotics) that reduce carnitine absorption or increase its excretion. Carnitine is used as a prescription to treat these deficiencies.

CAROTENOIDS

Carotenoids are the colorful plant pigments that give certain fruits and vegetables their yellow, orange, or red color. Some carotenoids, such as beta-carotene, alpha-carotene, and beta-cryptoxanthin, can be converted into vitamin A in the body. Other carotenoids, such as lycopene, lutein, and zeaxanthin, cannot be made into vitamin A by the body. More than 600 different carotenoids have been identified. Carotenoids are powerful protectors against cancer and heart disease. All carotenoids are antioxidants.

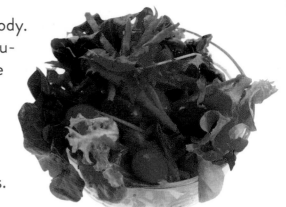

CHLORINE

Chlorine is an important regulator of body systems, such as water balance, acid-base balance, and fluid pressure. For example, this mineral is part of hydrochloric acid, needed in the stomach for digestion. The acidity it creates ensures proper absorption of food and reduces the growth of harmful bacteria.

There is no RDA for chlorine. Regular table salt is 60 percent chlorine, as chloride. This source, along with the salt that occurs naturally in foods, provides all the chlorine that's needed. Even a diet restricted in sodium can supply adequate amounts of chlorine.

A chlorine deficiency is not likely because chlorine is so prevalent in foods, but it can happen under certain circumstances. For example, several years ago some infant formula was processed without chlorine. Children fed this formula as their sole food source developed chlorine deficiencies.

CHOLINE

Choline is a substance found in most animal tissues. It can exist by itself or as part of another substance. For example, it can be found in lecithin, a waxy material in the protective myelin sheath that surrounds nerve fibers. It can also exist as part of the neurotransmitter acetylcholine, a substance essential for the transmission of impulses through the nervous system.

Sources of Choline

Many foods contain choline. Egg yolks, meat, fish, poultry, and dairy products are good sources of choline. Cruciferous vegetables and certain beans are also rich in choline. Other dietary sources of choline include nuts, seeds, and whole grains.

Some multivitamin-mineral supplements contain choline, often in the form of choline bitartrate, phosphatidylcholine, or lecithin. Dietary supplements with only choline are also available. Under normal circumstances, choline and lecithin supplements are not necessary because the body manufactures choline.

Recommended Intakes for Choline

No Recommended Dietary Allowances (RDAs) have been established for choline, but Adequate Intakes (AIs) and Tolerable Upper Intake Levels (ULs) have been set. The Tolerable Upper Intake Level (UL) is the maximum daily intake unlikely to cause adverse health effects. The AIs and ULs for choline are shown on the next page.

TOLERABLE UPPER INTAKE LEVELS (ULs) FOR CHOLINE

LIFE STAGE GROUP	MILLIGRAMS PER DAY
Infants 0–12 months	Not established
Children 1–8 years	1,000 mg
Children 9–13 years	2,000 mg
Teens 14–18 years	3,000 mg
Adults 19+ years	3,500 mg
Pregnant and breastfeeding teens 14–18 years	3,000 mg
Pregnant and breastfeeding women 19+ years	3,500 mg

ADEQUATE INTAKES (AIs) FOR CHOLINE

LIFE STAGE GROUP	MILLIGRAMS PER DAY
Infants 0–6 months	125 mg
Infants 7–12 months	150 mg
Children 1–3 years	200 mg
Children 4–8 years	250 mg
Children 9–13 years	375 mg
Teen boys 14–18 years	550 mg
Teen girls 14–18 years	400 mg
Men 19+ years	550 mg
Women 19+ years	425 mg
Pregnant teens and women	450 mg
Breastfeeding teens and women	550 mg

Deficiency of Choline

Most Americans don't get the recommended amounts of choline. However, few people in the U.S. have choline deficiency. One reason might be that the body can make some choline. Pregnant women, people with certain genetic conditions, and people being fed intravenously are more likely to have trouble getting sufficient choline. If choline levels drop too low, a condition called nonalcoholic fatty liver disease can occur.

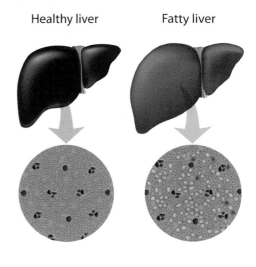

Healthy liver   Fatty liver

Choline and Health

There may be a link between low intakes of choline and the risk of developing nonalcoholic fatty liver disease, a condition in which fat builds up in the liver of people who do not drink excessive amounts of alcohol.

CHROMIUM

Chromium is part of the glucose tolerance factor (GTF) that regulates the actions of insulin—the hormone necessary for glucose metabolism. In chromium-deficient people, insulin doesn't function properly. In such cases, chromium supplements can improve the body's ability to handle glucose. Chromium is also important in the metabolism of fats and carbohydrates.

Sources of Chromium

Chromium is an essential mineral not made by the body—it must be obtained from the diet. A diet rich in refined carbohydrates such as sugar increases the need for chromium. And the more refined and processed foods are, the less chromium they contain.

Brewer's yeast and wheat germ are rich in chromium. Other sources include whole grains, meats, poultry, cheese and other dairy products, seafood, broccoli, and eggs.

Chromium supplements have become increasingly popular. They are sold as single-ingredient supplements and in combination supplements, especially those marketed for weight loss and performance enhancement. And though supplements may improve some people's chromium nutrition, they will not magically melt away pounds as some advertisements imply.

Recommended Intakes for Chromium

There is no established RDA for chromium. However, AIs were developed based on average intakes of chromium from food as found in several studies. The AIs are generally set at a level that healthy people typically consume. (The AIs for chromium are shown on the next page.) Women who are pregnant or breastfeeding need higher amounts. If you have diabetes or glucose intolerance, consult with a physician before taking supplements. Although they might benefit your condition, they might also alter your need for medication.

Adequate Intakes (AIs) for Chromium

LIFE STAGE GROUP	MICROGRAMS PER DAY
Infants 0–6 months	0.2 mcg
Infants 7–12 months	5.5 mcg
Children 1–3 years	11 mcg
Children 4–8 years	15 mcg
Boys 9–13 years	25 mcg
Girls 9–13 years	21 mcg
Boys 14–18 years	35 mcg
Girls 14–18 years	24 mcg
Men 19–50 years	35 mcg
Women 19–50 years	25 mcg
Men 51+ years	30 mcg
Women 51+ years	20 mcg
Pregnant teens 14–18 years	29 mcg
Pregnant women 19–50 years	30 mcg
Breastfeeding teens 14–18 years	44 mcg
Breastfeeding women 19–50 years	45 mcg

Chromium Deficiency and Excess

Chromium deficiency may be seen as impaired glucose tolerance. It occurs in older people with type 2 diabetes and in infants with protein-calorie malnutrition. A chromium supplement may help, but should not substitute other treatment.

Few serious adverse effects have been linked to high intakes of chromium because of the low absorption and high excretion rates.

Chromium and Health

There is a great deal of interest in the possibility that chromium supplements may help treat impaired glucose tolerance and type 2 diabetes, but the research to date is inconclusive.

Researchers are also studying whether chromium supplements can help treat diabetes, lower blood lipid levels, promote weight loss, and improve body composition.

COBALT

Cobalt is an organic substance needed in very small amounts. As part of vitamin B_{12}, cobalt plays a major role in the body's metabolic processes. There is no RDA for cobalt because it is usually obtained from vitamin B_{12}. A cobalt deficiency can lead to anemia. Too much cobalt can lead to a greater than normal number of red blood cells. See the full vitamin B_{12} profile on page 168.

COENZYME Q10

Coenzyme Q10, or CoQ10, is an antioxidant that is necessary for proper cell function. Cells use CoQ10 to make the energy they need to grow and stay healthy.

Fish, meats, and whole grains provide small amounts of CoQ10, but not enough to significantly increase levels in the body. Levels of CoQ10 decrease as you get older.

CoQ10 may stimulate the immune system and protect the heart from damage caused by certain chemotherapy drugs. CoQ10 supplements may also benefit some people with cardiovascular disorders.

CoQ10 supplements are generally well tolerated and have mild side effects. However, CoQ10 can interact with other medications. CoQ10 may change the way body uses warfarin (a blood thinner) and insulin. Other drugs may decrease the effects of CoQ10. Talk with your health care provider before starting a CoQ10 supplement.

COPPER

Copper helps the body absorb and use iron. It's part of several enzymes that help form hemoglobin (the oxygen-carrying pigment in red blood cells) and collagen (a connective-tissue protein found in skin and tendons). Copper also helps keep the immune system, blood vessels, nerves, and bones healthy.

Sources of Copper

Good sources of copper include oysters and other shellfish, whole grains, potatoes, beans, nuts, and liver. Prunes and other dried fruits, dark leafy greens, cocoa, yeast, and black pepper are also sources of copper.

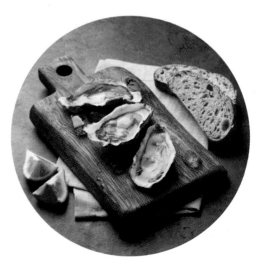

Recommended Dietary Allowances (RDAs) for Copper

LIFE STAGE GROUP	MICROGRAMS PER DAY
Infants 0–6 months	200 mcg*
Infants 7–12 months	220 mcg*
Children 1–3 years	340 mcg
Children 4–8 years	440 mcg
Children 9–13 years	700 mcg
Teens 14–18 years	890 mcg
Adults 19+ years	900 mcg
Pregnant teens and women	1,000 mcg
Breastfeeding teens and women	1,300 mcg

*Adequate Intake (AI)

Tolerable Upper Intake Levels (ULs) for Copper

LIFE STAGE GROUP	MICROGRAMS PER DAY
Infants 0–12 months	Not established
Children 1–3 years	1,000 mcg
Children 4–8 years	3,000 mcg
Children 9–13 years	5,000 mcg
Teens 14–18 years	8,000 mcg
Adults 19+ years	10,000 mcg
Pregnant and breastfeeding teens 14–18 years	8,000 mcg
Pregnant and breastfeeding women 19+ years	10,000 mcg

Copper Deficiency and Excess

A dietary deficiency of copper is very rare but has occurred in severely malnourished children, disrupting their growth and metabolism. It can also occur in infants born prematurely because copper isn't usually transferred from the mother to the fetus until the last few weeks of pregnancy. Lack of copper may lead to anemia and osteoporosis.

An excessive intake of copper, which has been reported to occur after water was stored in copper tanks, may cause headaches, dizziness, nausea, and vomiting. Excessive copper consumption can cause gastro-intestinal distress and liver damage.

Copper and Health

Several rare genetic diseases, including Wilson disease, Menkes disease, and Indian childhood cirrhosis, are associated with the improper utilization of copper in the body. Menkes disease (kinky hair syndrome) is a very rare copper metabolism disorder that occurs primarily in male infants.

Children who inherit the gene for Wilson disease cannot get rid of excess copper. It accumulates in certain organs in their bodies, especially the eyes, brain, liver, and kidneys. The increased copper in these tissues can lead to hepatitis, kidney problems, brain disorders, and other problems. It's treated with a copper-free diet and medication designed to bind with the copper, rendering it harmless.

ECHINACEA

The roots and sometimes the leaves of this beautiful sunflower family member (*Echinacea purpurea*) are used fresh or dried to make teas, squeezed juice, extracts, capsules and tablets, and preparations for external use. Several species of echinacea are used in dietary supplements.

Echinacea has been a traditional medicine used widely to treat colds, flu, bronchitis, and certain types of infections. While many studies have examined echinacea and the common cold, much less research has been done on the use of echinacea for other health purposes.

History

This showy perennial was used by Native Americans and adopted by early settlers as a medicine. Members of the medical profession in early America relied heavily on echinacea, but it fell from favor with the advent of pharmaceutical medicine and antibiotics. Many physicians are rediscovering the benefits of echinacea today.

Long used for infectious diseases and poor immune function, echinacea extractions are also used today to help treat cancer, chronic fatigue syndrome, and AIDS. Research has shown echinacea stimulates the body's natural immune function. It also increases both the number and the activity of white blood cells, raises the level of interferon, and stimulates blood cells to engulf invading microbes. Echinacea also increases the production of substances the body produces naturally to fight cancers and disease.

Besides its use as an immune stimulant, echinacea is recommended for individuals with recurring boils and as an antidote for snakebites.

Sources of Echinacea

There are many different echinacea products on the market. They may contain different species of plants, use different parts of the plant, be manufactured differently, and have other ingredients in addition to echinacea. Keep in mind that most of these echinacea products have not been tested in people.

Echinacea Uses

Echinacea is not terribly tasty in a tea. For this reason, echinacea is most often taken as tincture or as pills. However, teas and tinctures appear to be more effective than the powdered herb in capsules. If you take the capsules, first break them open and put them in a little warm water; then drink the water. Most herbalists recommend large and frequent doses of echinacea at the onset of a cold, flu, sinus infection, bladder infection, or other illness.

For acute infection: Take 1 dropper full of tincture every one to three hours, or 1 to 2 capsules every three to four hours for the first day or two; then reduce the dosage.

For a chronic infectious problem: Take echinacea three times a day for several weeks and then abstain for several weeks before continuing again.

FLAVONOIDS

Flavonoids are health-protective substances found in the colorful skins of fruits and vegetables as well as in beverages such as tea, red wine, and fruit juices. Their health benefits are similar to those of antioxidants.

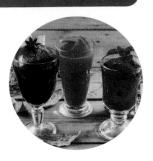

FLUORIDE

Fluoride is an essential trace mineral found in bones, teeth, and body fluids. If fluoride is available when bones and teeth develop, it's incorporated into their structures, making teeth more resistant to decay and bones more resistant to osteoporosis. Fluoride also maintains the structure of bones and teeth after they are formed.

Sources of Fluoride

Water is the most common source of fluoride in the diet. Food prepared in fluoridated water also contains fluoride. Most seafood contains fluoride since there is natural sodium fluoride in the ocean. Tea is a surprisingly good source as well. A cup of tea provides about 0.2 milligrams of fluoride.

Research shows that people who live in areas where the drinking water contains less than one part per million of fluoride have more dental decay and osteoporosis. In many areas of the country, water is fluoridated to a level of one part per million—the optimal level. Studies clearly show that children raised in such areas have 50 percent fewer cavities than children who do not drink fluoridated water.

In areas where the natural fluoride concentration in the water is high (two to eight parts per million), the enamel on children's teeth may become mottled (spotted)—a condition called fluorosis. The condition doesn't seem to be harmful; in fact, mottled teeth are very resistant to decay.

Recommended Intakes for Fluoride

There are no RDAs for fluoride, but there are Adequate Intakes (AIs) and Tolerable Upper Intake Levels (ULs).

ADEQUATE INTAKES (AIs) FOR FLUORIDE

LIFE STAGE GROUP	MILLIGRAMS PER DAY
Infants 0–6 months	0.01 mg
Infants 7–12 months	0.5 mg
Children 1–3 years	0.7 mg
Children 4–8 years	1.0 mg
Children 9–13 years	2.0 mg
Teen boys 14–18 years	3.0 mg
Males 19+ years	4.0 mg
Females 14+ years	3.0 mg
Pregnant and breastfeeding women	3.0 mg

TOLERABLE UPPER INTAKE LEVELS (ULs) FOR FLUORIDE

LIFE STAGE GROUP	MILLIGRAMS PER DAY
Infants 0–6 months	0.7 mg
Infants 7–12 months	0.9 mg
Children 1–3 years	1.3 mg
Children 4–8 years	2.2 mg
Males 9+ years	10 mg
Females 9+ years	10 mg
Pregnant and breastfeeding women	10 mg

FOLATE (VITAMIN B9)

Folate refers to the various forms of the same B vitamin. Folate is naturally present in some foods, added to others, and available as a dietary supplement. Folate occurs naturally in foods such as leafy green vegetables, fruits, and dried beans and peas. Folic acid is the synthetic form of folate used in supplements and fortified foods.

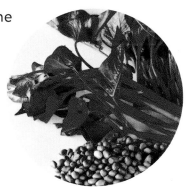

History

The discovery of folate was closely tied to the discovery of vitamin B_{12}. These two vitamins work together in several important biological reactions. A deficiency of either vitamin results in a condition known as megaloblastic or macrocytic (large-cell) anemia.

In 1930, researcher Lucy Wills and her colleagues reported that yeast contained a substance that could cure macrocytic anemia in pregnant women. But it wasn't until the early 1940s that folate was finally isolated and identified.

Functions of Folate

Folate functions as a coenzyme during many reactions in the body. It has an important role in making new cells, because it helps form the genetic material DNA (deoxyribonucleic acid) and RNA (ribonucleic acid). DNA carries and RNA transmits the genetic information that acts as the blueprint for cell production.

We especially need folate when new cells are manufactured. This function of folate helps to explain why the vitamin is necessary for normal growth and development, and why anemia occurs when there's not enough. The body makes large numbers of red blood cells each day to replace those it destroys. DNA is essential for this process; therefore, folate is as well.

Sources of Folate

Green leafy vegetables, such as broccoli, spinach, and asparagus, are rich in folate. (Take care not to overcook vegetables, or the folate may be lost.) Seeds, liver, and dried peas and beans are other good sources. Orange juice is a good source of folate because it contains the most readily absorbed form of the vitamin. It also contains vitamin C, and vitamin C helps preserve folate.

Folic acid (a form of folate) is available in multivitamins (generally at a dose of 400 mcg) and prenatal vitamins. Folic acid is especially important for women who are pregnant, as it can help prevent major birth defects of the baby's brain or spine. Folic acid is also available in B-complex dietary supplements and in standalone supplements.

Recommended Intakes for Folate

The RDAs for folate are listed in micrograms (mcg) of dietary folate equivalents (DFEs). The Food and Nutrition Board developed dietary folate equivalents (DFEs) to reflect the easier absorption of folic acid in supplements and fortified foods compared with folate found naturally in foods, which is absorbed only about half as well.

> 1 MCG DFE = 1 MICROGRAM (MCG) FOOD FOLATE
>
> 1 MCG DFE = 0.6 MCG FOLIC ACID FROM FORTIFIED FOODS OR SUPPLEMENTS CONSUMED WITH FOODS
>
> 1 MCG DFE = 0.5 MCG FOLIC ACID FROM SUPPLEMENTS TAKEN ON AN EMPTY STOMACH

The RDA for folate is 400 mcg DFE for adults. Pregnant women require 600 mcg DFE because so many new cells are being made. Women who are breastfeeding require 500 mcg DFE. Note that the Tolerable Upper Intake Levels (ULs) on the next page are for folic acid from dietary supplements and fortified foods, not for folate from food sources. No UL was established for folate from food because no adverse effects have been reported from high intakes.

Recommended Dietary Allowances (RDAs) for Folate

LIFE STAGE GROUP	MCG DFE PER DAY
Infants 0–6 months	65 mcg DFE*
Infants 7–12 months	80 mcg DFE*
Children 1–3 years	150 mcg DFE
Children 4–8 years	200 mcg DFE
Children 9–13 years	300 mcg DFE
Teens 14–18 years	400 mcg DFE
Adults 19+ years	400 mcg DFE
Pregnant teens and women	600 mcg DFE
Breastfeeding teens and women	500 mcg DFE

*Adequate Intake (AI)

Tolerable Upper Intake Levels (ULs) for Folic Acid

LIFE STAGE GROUP	MICROGRAMS PER DAY
Infants 0–12 months	Not established
Children 1–3 years	300 mcg
Children 4–8 years	400 mcg
Children 9–13 years	600 mcg
Teens 14–18 years	800 mcg
Adults 19+ years	1,000 mcg
Pregnant and breastfeeding teens 14–18 years	800 mcg
Pregnant and breastfeeding women 19+ years	1,000 mcg

Deficiency of Folate

Folate deficiency is relatively rare in the United States. Most people get enough folate. However, certain groups are at risk of insufficient folate intakes. These groups include women of childbearing age, non-Hispanic black women, people with alcohol dependence, and people with disorders that lower nutrient absorption.

Some medications can interfere with the body's ability to use this vitamin. These medications include aspirin, oral contraceptives, and drugs used to treat convulsions, psoriasis, and cancer. In addition, abuse of alcohol can damage the intestine so that less folate is absorbed.

Insufficient folate can result in megaloblastic anemia, which causes weakness, fatigue, trouble concentrating, irritability, headache, heart palpitations, and shortness of breath. Folate deficiency can also cause open sores on the tongue and inside the mouth as well as changes in the color of skin, hair, or fingernails.

Women who don't get enough folate are at risk of having babies with neural tube defects, such as spina bifida. Folate deficiency can also increase the likelihood of having a premature or low-birth-weight baby.

Experts now emphasize the importance of folate supplementation in the very early stages of pregnancy because the vitamin plays an important role in early fetal development. Because folate is so important at a time when many women might not even know they are pregnant, women planning to conceive—and any women capable of becoming pregnant—should be sure they are getting enough folate.

Folate Use and Misuse

Doctors prescribe folate supplements if they diagnose a folate deficiency and have ruled out a vitamin B_{12} deficiency. Excessive intake of folate may actually mask a deficiency of vitamin B_{12} or an underlying case of pernicious anemia. Large doses of folate cause the blood to appear normal, which, in turn, may delay diagnosis and treatment of vitamin B_{12} deficiency, resulting in serious, irreversible damage to the nervous system. The longer the delay, the more serious the damage.

No adverse effects have been reported due to high intakes of folate from food sources. Folic acid supplements can, however, interact with medications used to treat epilepsy, psychiatric diseases, cancer, and ulcerative colitis.

FOLIC ACID (VITAMIN B9)

Folic acid is a form of the B vitamin folate. It helps the body make healthy new cells. Everyone needs folic acid. For women who may get pregnant, it is especially important. Getting enough folic acid before and during pregnancy can prevent serious birth defects. Folic acid is found in dietary supplements and fortified foods, such as breads, pastas, and cereals. See the full folate profile for more information.

GARLIC

Garlic (*Allium sativum*) belongs to the lily family and is one of the most extensively researched and widely used of all plants. Its actions are diverse and affect nearly every body tissue and system. Lots of people include garlic in their daily diet for health reasons, while many others eat it because they love its pungent flavor.

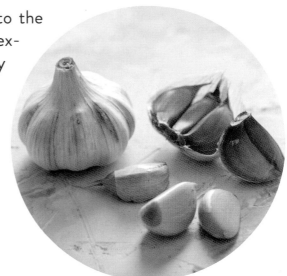

Functions of Garlic

As an antimicrobial, garlic seems to have a broad action. It displays antibiotic, antifungal, and antiviral properties. You may add garlic liberally to foods during the winter months to help prevent colds, or eat garlic at the first hint of a cold, cough, or flu. Garlic also reduces congestion and may help people with bronchitis to expel mucus.

Garlic contains a large number of rather unique sulfur-containing compounds, which are credited with many of this herb's medicinal actions. Did you ever wonder why garlic bulbs on your kitchen counter don't have a strong odor until you cut or crush them? That's because an enzyme in garlic promotes conversion of the chemical compound alliin to the odorous allicin. Allicin and other sulfur compounds are potent antimicrobials and are thought to have blood purifying and, possibly, anticancer effects.

Some studies show that certain groups of people who eat more garlic may be less likely to develop certain cancers, including cancers of the stomach, colon, esophagus, pancreas, and breast. Garlic in dietary supplement form, however, does not appear to help reduce the risk of these cancers. The National Cancer Institute (part of the National Institutes of Health) recognizes garlic as one of several vegetables with potential anticancer properties, but does not recommend garlic dietary supplements for cancer prevention.

Garlic appears to lowers blood pressure by relaxing vein and artery walls. This action helps keep platelets from clumping together and improves blood flow, thereby reducing the risk of stroke. Evidence about whether garlic lowers blood cholesterol levels is conflicting. If it does, the effect is relatively small. And levels of LDL (low-density lipoprotein, or "bad" cholesterol) may not be reduced at all.

Use of Garlic

Garlic is available fresh, dried, powdered, and tinctured. In health food stores, garlic appears primarily in capsule form or combined in tablets with other herbs. Since garlic's antibiotic properties depend on odorous allicin, deodorized garlic preparations are not effective for this use. The label of such products may identify them as having a particular "allicin content," but they remain ineffective as antibiotics. Of course, the tastiest way to get your dose of garlic is to add it liberally to your diet.

The World Health Organization's guidelines for general health promotion suggest that adults get a daily dose of 2 to 5 grams of fresh garlic (approximately one clove), 0.4 to 1.2 grams of dried garlic powder, 2 to 5 milligrams of garlic oil, 300 to 1,000 milligrams of garlic extract, or other formulations that are equal to 2 to 5 milligrams of allicin.

When to Avoid Garlic

Garlic acts as a natural blood thinner and should be avoided by pregnant women, people about to undergo surgery, and people taking blood thinners.

Garlic can interfere with the effectiveness of several prescription drugs, especially the HIV medication saquinavir.

Garlic occasionally causes allergic reactions ranging from mild irritation to potentially life-threatening problems. Ingestion of fresh garlic bulbs, extracts, or oil on an empty stomach may occasionally cause heartburn, nausea, vomiting, and diarrhea.

People who are prone to stomach conditions, such as ulcers, should avoid garlic, as it can exacerbate the condition or cause new ones.

GINGER

This botanical and popular spice (*Zingiber officinale*) is native to Southeast Asia but is now readily available in the United States. Fresh ginger root is a staple in Asian cooking. Dried and powdered, it's used in medicine.

Therapeutic Value

Ginger has long been used for nausea and vomiting. As a stomach-calming agent, ginger reduces gas, bloating, and indigestion, and aids in the body's use and absorption of other nutrients and medicines. Ginger may help relieve pregnancy-related nausea and vomiting. Ginger may help to control nausea related to cancer chemotherapy when used with conventional anti-nausea medication. It's not clear if ginger is helpful for post-surgery nausea, motion sickness, rheumatoid arthritis, or osteoarthritis.

When to Avoid Ginger

People with fevers or menopausal hot flashes should avoid ginger since it can warm and raise body temperature slightly.

Although ginger can help morning sickness, those with a history of miscarriage should avoid it. Since ginger stimulates blood flow and thins the blood, promoting uterine bleeding is a concern.

Some people actually become nauseous if they consume a large quantity of ginger; for others, ginger relieves nausea. It is best to use ginger cautiously at first.

GINKGO

This stately deciduous tree produces male and female flowers on separate plants. Female plants produce orange-yellow fruits the size of large olives. In the fall its leaves turn gold. Found throughout the temperate world, ginkgo may be grown in many parts of the United States. It is cultivated extensively.

The ginkgo tree (*Ginkgo biloba*) is one of the oldest tree species on Earth. It is used to treat conditions associated with aging, including stroke, heart disease, impotence, deafness, ringing in the ears (tinnitus), blindness, and memory loss. In many studies, it helped people improve their concentration and memory. Ginkgo promotes the action of certain neurotransmitters, chemical compounds responsible for relaying nerve impulses in the brain. It is even undergoing investigation as a treatment for diabetes.

Ginkgo increases circulation, including blood flow to the brain, which may help improve memory. Several studies show it reduces the risk of heart attack and improves pain from blood clots (phlebitis) in the legs. Additional studies show that, in a large percentage of people, ginkgo helps impotence caused by narrowing of arteries that supply blood to the penis; macular degeneration of the eyes, a deterioration in vision that may be caused by narrowing of the blood vessels to the eye; and cochlear deafness, which is caused by decreased blood flow to the nerves involved in hearing.

Constituents in ginkgo are potent antioxidants with anti-inflammatory effects. A current scientific theory attributes many of the signs of aging and chronic disease to oxidation of cell membranes by substances called free radicals, which may arise from pollutants or from normal internal production of metabolic substances. Ginkgo counters destruction of cells due to oxidation. Scientists are also investigating ginkgo as a medicine that one day may help the body accept transplanted organs. Researchers also found it may help children with asthma.

The herb produces chemicals that interfere with a substance called platelet activation factor, PAF, which is involved in organ graft rejection, asthma attacks, and blood clots that lead to heart attacks and some strokes.

Ginkgo is made into tablets, capsules, extracts, teas, and cosmetics. For most healthy people, ginkgo is considered safe in recommended doses. Ginkgo may interact with some medications so talk with your health care provider before starting a ginkgo supplement.

Side effects of ginkgo include headache, stomach upset, and allergic skin reactions. Older people, people with a known bleeding risk, and pregnant women should be cautious about ginkgo possibly increasing the risk of bleeding.

GINSENG

Enthusiasm over ginseng began thousands of years ago in China, where the Asian species of ginseng, *Panax ginseng*, grows. Asian ginseng is one of several types of ginseng. Dietary supplements of Asian ginseng are used to stimulate the immune system; improve well-being, stamina, and concentration; slow aging; and relieve various health problems, including respiratory disorders, cardiovascular disorders, depression, and anxiety.

Therapeutic Value

Asian ginseng is used as a general tonic by modern Western herbalists as well as by traditional Chinese practitioners. It is thought to gently stimulate and strengthen the central nervous system in cases of fatigue, physical exertion, weakness from disease and injury, and prolonged emotional stress. Its most widespread use is among the elderly. It is reported to help control diabetes, improve blood pressure and heart action, and reduce mental confusion, headaches, and weakness among the elderly. Asian ginseng's affinity for the nervous system and its ability to promote relaxation makes it useful for stress-related conditions such as insomnia and anxiety.

Ginseng contains many chemical components called ginsenosides that are thought to contribute to the herb's health-related properties. Ginsenosides have been extensively studied and found to have numerous complex actions, including the following: They stimulate bone marrow production, stimulate the immune system, inhibit tumor growth, balance blood sugar, stabilize blood pressure, and detoxify the liver, among many other tonic effects. Ginseng also contains numerous other constituents, yet no one constituent has been identified as the most active. In fact, many of the individual constituents have been shown to have opposite actions. Like all plant medicine, the activity is due to the sum total of all the substances.

When to Avoid Ginseng

Ginseng is one of the better-researched plants, and short-term use of Asian ginseng in recommended amounts appears to be safe for most people. Due to hormonal activity, ginseng should be avoided during pregnancy. Some experts also recommend against ginseng's use by infants, children, and nursing mothers. Some cases of hypertension are aggravated by ginseng while others are improved; consult an herbalist, naturopathic physician, or other practitioner trained in the use of herbal medicine for the use of ginseng in hypertension.

HAWTHORN

Like many members of the rose family, hawthorn bears thorns as well as lovely, fragrant flowers and brightly pigmented berries high in vitamin C. As many as 900 species of hawthorn exist in North America, ranging from deciduous trees to thorny-branched shrubs. Hawthorn produces white flower clusters in May. The herb is native to Europe, with closely related species in North Africa and western Asia. It is often found in areas with hedges and deciduous woods.

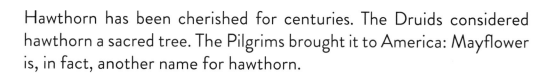

Hawthorn has been cherished for centuries. The Druids considered hawthorn a sacred tree. The Pilgrims brought it to America: Mayflower is, in fact, another name for hawthorn.

Hawthorn is an important herb for treating heart conditions. The berries and flowers contain several complex chemical constituents, including flavonoids such as anthocyanidins, which improve the strength of capillaries and reduce damage to blood vessels from oxidizing agents. Hawthorn's ability to dilate blood vessels, enhancing circulation, makes it useful for treating angina, atherosclerosis, high and low blood pressure, and elevated cholesterol levels.

Many clinical studies have demonstrated its effectiveness for such conditions—with the use of hawthorn, the heart requires less oxygen when under stress. Heart action is normalized and becomes stronger and more efficient. Hawthorn also helps balance the heart's rhythm and is prescribed for arrhythmias and heart palpitations by European physicians. Although it affects the heart somewhat like the medication digitalis, hawthorn does not have a cumulative effect on the heart.

Hawthorn extracts from the leaf, flower, or berry are sold in the form of capsules, tablets, or liquids. Hawthorn is generally considered safe and may be used for long periods.

Do not self-medicate with hawthorn. Consult your health care provider before taking hawthorn, especially if you take prescription heart medication. Hawthorn may intensify the effects of these drugs.

INOSITOL

Inositol is a water-soluble vitamin-like substance that is similar to the B-complex vitamins. Liver, wheat germ, citrus fruits, and meats are rich sources of inositol. Of the nine related compounds that are collectively called inositol, the only one that is considered important to plants and animals is myo-inositol. Researchers don't yet completely understand myo-inosital's function, but it is believed to aid in the metabolism of fats. While the term "inositol" is often used with dietary supplements, it usually only refers to myo-inositol.

IODINE

Iodine is a trace element naturally present in some foods, added to others, and available in the form of supplements. Iodine is an important component of thyroid hormones, which control energy metabolism in the body. Thyroid hormones are also required for proper bone and brain development during pregnancy and infancy.

Sources of Iodine

Saltwater seafood is a primary source of iodine. Iodized salt, in use since 1924, is another rich source. One teaspoon of iodized salt provides 260 micrograms (mcg) of iodine. The amount of iodine in vegetables and grains varies according to how much is present in the soil where they are grown. In certain regions of the world, this amount is less than optimal.

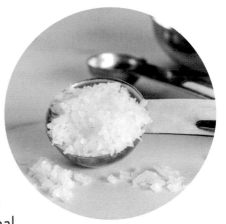

In the United States, the need for iodized salt is not as great as it was 60 years ago. Thanks to refrigerated trucks, most of the country gets produce from coastal regions where soil is rich in iodine. Iodine deficiency is a concern only in isolated areas where all the food eaten is locally grown.

Dairy equipment is sometimes disinfected with iodine-containing compounds, and dairy cattle are given iodine-containing feed. Both contribute to an increasing amount of iodine in milk and dairy products. Iodine is also in dough conditioners used by bakeries, in food colorings, and even in polluted air.

Iodine is also available in dietary supplements, typically in the form of potassium iodide or sodium iodide. Iodine is included in many multivitamin-mineral supplements. Iodine-containing kelp (a seaweed) dietary supplements are available as well.

RECOMMENDED DIETARY ALLOWANCES (RDAS) FOR IODINE

LIFE STAGE GROUP	MICROGRAMS PER DAY
Infants 0–6 months	110 mcg*
Infants 7–12 months	130 mcg*
Children 1–8 years	90 mcg
Children 9–13 years	120 mcg
Teens 14–18 years	150 mcg
Adults 19+ years	150 mcg
Pregnant teens and women	220 mcg
Breastfeeding teens and women	290 mcg

*Adequate Intake (AI)

TOLERABLE UPPER INTAKE LEVELS (ULS) FOR IODINE

LIFE STAGE GROUP	MICROGRAMS PER DAY
Infants 0–12 months	Not established
Children 1–3 years	200 mcg
Children 4–8 years	300 mcg
Children 9–13 years	600 mcg
Teens 14–18 years	900 mcg
Adults 19+ years	1,100 mcg
Pregnant and breastfeeding teens 14–18 years	900 mcg
Pregnant and breastfeeding women 19+ years	1,100 mcg

Deficiency of Iodine

Iodine deficiency is rare in the United States today, but still a problem in other parts of the world. Certain groups are more likely to have insufficient iodine intakes, including people who don't use iodized salt, pregnant women, people who eat foods grown in iodine-deficient soils, and people who don't get much iodine and also eat foods containing goitrogens.

A deficiency of iodine can cause the thyroid gland to greatly enlarge—a condition known as goiter. The thyroid gland, which is normally about the size of a lima bean, can sometimes become as large as a person's head. A deficiency of thyroid hormones can result in mental and physical sluggishness, slowed heart rate, weight gain, constipation, and increased sleep needs (14–16 hours a day). In pregnancy, the results of iodine deficiency are more serious. The baby of an iodine-deficient mother may have stunted physical and mental development—a condition known as cretinism.

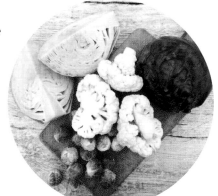

Substances known as goitrogens induce goiter when iodine intake is low. Cabbage, Brussels sprouts, cauliflower, turnips, and peanuts contain these substances. However, since heat destroys goitrogens, the potential dangers exist only if large amounts of these foods are eaten raw.

Iodine Use and Misuse

Iodine supplements (including iodized salt) are used to prevent and treat iodine deficiencies and their consequences, including goiter and some thyroid disorders. Taking iodine by mouth can improve thyroid storm, a rare but potentially life-threatening complication of hyperthyroidism (overactive thyroid gland), and lumps on the thyroid called thyroid nodules.

Iodine is also used for radiation emergencies to protect the thyroid gland against radioactive iodides. Nuclear accidents can release radioactive iodine into the environment, increasing the risk of thyroid cancer in exposed individuals. Children and people with iodine deficiency are especially at risk of developing thyroid cancer. The FDA has approved potassium iodide as a thyroid-blocking agent to reduce the risk of thyroid cancer in radiation emergencies. However, potassium iodine should not be used for general protection against radiation.

Getting too much iodine can cause some of the same symptoms as iodine deficiency, including goiter (an enlarged thyroid gland). Very large doses of iodine (many grams, for example) can cause burning in the mouth and throat, abdominal pain, diarrhea, vomiting, weak pulse, and many other side effects.

Iodine can also interact with several medications, including anti-thyroid drugs, ACE inhibitors for high blood pressure, and potassium-sparing diuretics. Talk with your health care provider before starting any iodine supplements.

IRON

Most of the body's iron resides in the hemoglobin of red blood cells—the pigment that makes these blood cells appear red. Hemoglobin carries oxygen to cells and transports carbon dioxide from cells. Iron is also essential to enzymes involved in energy release, cholesterol metabolism, immune function, and connective-tissue production.

Sources of Iron

Iron in food comes in two forms—heme iron and nonheme iron. Lean meat and seafood are the richest dietary sources of heme iron. Sources of nonheme iron include nuts, beans, vegetables, and fortified grain products. Meat, seafood, and poultry have both heme and nonheme iron.

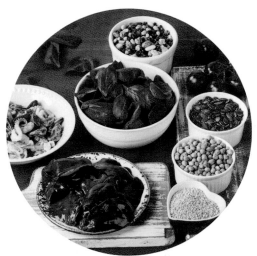

Other food sources of iron include white beans, lentils, spinach, kidney beans, peas, dark chocolate, tofu, and raisins.

Nonheme iron from plant sources is better absorbed when eaten with meat, poultry, seafood, and vitamin C-rich foods (e.g., citrus fruits, strawberries, sweet peppers, tomatoes, broccoli).

Iron is available in many multivitamin-mineral supplements and in iron-only supplements. The iron in supplements is often in the form of ferrous sulfate, ferric citrate, ferrous gluconate, or ferric sulfate. Dietary supplements that contain iron should be kept out of the reach of children, as accidental overdose of iron is a leading cause of fatal poisoning in young children.

Recommended Intakes for Iron

The table on the next page shows the RDAs for non-vegetarians. Vegetarians who do not eat meat, poultry, or seafood need 1.8 times more iron than people who eat meat because the body doesn't absorb nonheme iron in plant foods as well as heme iron in animal foods.

Recommended Dietary Allowances (RDAs) for Iron

LIFE STAGE GROUP	MILLIGRAMS PER DAY
Infants 0–6 months	0.27 mg*
Infants 7–12 months	11 mg
Children 1–3 years	7 mg
Children 4–8 years	10 mg
Children 9–13 years	8 mg
Teen boys 14–18 years	11 mg
Teen girls 14–18 years	15 mg
Men 19–50 years	8 mg
Women 19–50 years	18 mg
Adults 51+ years	8 mg
Pregnant teens and women	27 mg
Breastfeeding teens 14–18 years	10 mg
Breastfeeding women 19+ years	9 mg

*Adequate Intake (AI)

Deficiency of Iron

While most Americans get enough iron, certain groups are more likely to have insufficient intakes of iron. These include teens and women with heavy periods; pregnant teens and women; infants, especially premature babies or babies with low birth weight; frequent blood donors; people who don't eat meat, poultry, or seafood; and people with cancer, heart failure, or gastrointestinal disorders that interfere with nutrient absorption.

Iron deficiency anemia may not cause obvious symptoms at first. But as the body uses its stored iron and the anemia worsens, the signs and symptoms intensify. Tiredness and lack of energy; chest pain, heart palpitations, or shortness of breath; headache, dizziness, or lightheadedness; poor memory and concentration; and sore tongue are some of the symptoms of iron deficiency anemia. For people who are anemic, even mild exercise can cause chest pain. Mild iron deficiency, even without anemia, may cause learning problems in schoolchildren. Pica, an abnormal desire to eat nonfood substances such as clay, chalk, ashes, or laundry starch (none of which contains iron), sometimes accompanies iron deficiency. That's because the eating of such nonfoods may interfere with iron absorption and may be a factor contributing to the anemia.

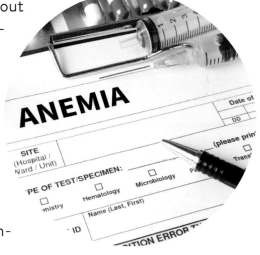

Iron Use and Misuse

To treat an iron deficiency, you need iron supplements in conjunction with an iron-rich diet. Iron is available in both a ferrous and ferric form (the Latin name for iron is *Ferrum*, hence the symbol Fe). Iron in the ferrous form is better absorbed than ferric iron. When you read labels of iron supplements, you should note that the number of milligrams for each tablet refers both to the iron it contains and the carrier to which it's bound. For example, the label may state, "Each tablet provides 200 mg of ferrous fumarate, which yields 67 mg of elemental iron." The amount of elemental iron is what you should consider.

Some people don't tolerate iron supplements well and may develop side effects such as heartburn, nausea, stomachache, constipation, or diarrhea. Taking the supplement with food can eliminate or minimize these symptoms. You can also gradually work up to the desired dose or divide the high dose into several small doses. Do not worry if your stool appears dark or black. It's just some of the unabsorbed iron.

In healthy people, the intestines control the amount of iron that's absorbed. The body increases its rate of iron absorption if reserves are low. And when the body becomes saturated with iron, the rate of absorption decreases. If the intestines do not or cannot properly perform this regulatory function—as can happen from excessive and prolonged alcohol intake—the body can absorb toxic quantities.

A certain percentage of the population suffers from hemochromatosis, a hereditary disease in which the body absorbs too much iron and deposits it in body tissues. Unfortunately, symptoms of this condition only appear after significant and irreversible damage occurs. They include weakness, weight loss, change in skin color, abdominal pain, loss of sex drive, and the onset of diabetes. Heart, liver, and joints may become impaired as well. This disease affects men more often than women. The treatment for this disease involves the removal of excess iron in the body.

Iron poisoning is the most common accidental poisoning in young children. Excess iron can be fatal. All supplements should be kept out of the reach of children.

LIPOIC ACID

Lipoic acid is a naturally occurring compound that is synthesized in small amounts by plants and animals, including humans. Lipoic acid has a coenzyme function similar to that of the vitamin thiamin. Alpha-lipoic acid supplements are commonly taken for diabetes and nerve-related symptoms of diabetes. Yeast, liver, kidney, spinach, broccoli, and potatoes are good sources of alpha-lipoic acid.

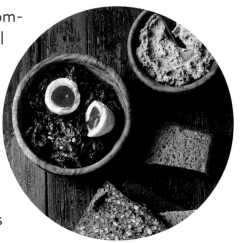

LUTEIN

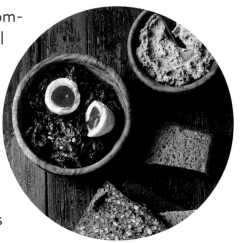

Lutein is a pigment found in foods that are bright yellow, orange, and green. Lutein is a carotenoid related to beta-carotene and vitamin A. This carotenoid is linked to a reduced risk of age-related macular degeneration and cataracts. Food sources of lutein include spinach, broccoli, kale, orange peppers, corn, kiwifruit, grapes, orange juice, zucchini, and squash. Lutein is also included in many multivitamin-mineral supplements.

LYCOPENE

Lycopene is a powerful antioxidant that gives numerous foods their red color and is especially abundant in tomatoes. It is thought to help protect cells from damage. Food sources of lycopene include tomatoes, tomato juice, ketchup, watermelons, red oranges, pink grapefruits, apricots, rosehips, and guavas. Lycopene can also be found in dietary supplements.

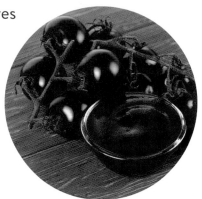

MAGNESIUM

Magnesium is a mineral the body needs for healthy nerves, muscles, and bones. Magnesium is a vital part of the mineral structure of bones and teeth. As with calcium, bones act as a reservoir for magnesium so that it will be available when needed.

Magnesium plays a role in protein synthesis, muscle relaxation, and energy release. It also triggers important metabolic reactions, including calcium metabolism. The parathyroid hormone needs magnesium to function normally; this regulates blood calcium levels.

Sources of Magnesium

Magnesium is found in many foods, particularly green leafy vegetables. This is because magnesium is part of chlorophyll, the pigment in plants that makes them green and fosters photosynthesis. Some breakfast cereals are fortified with magnesium. Other sources of magnesium are nuts and seeds; peas and beans; dairy products; whole grains; and chocolate. Hard water also contains significant amounts of magnesium.

FOOD SOURCES OF MAGNESIUM

FOOD	QUANTITY	MILLIGRAMS
Navy beans, cooked	1 cup	108 mg
Black-eyed peas, cooked	1 cup	91 mg
Almonds, dry roasted	1 ounce	80 mg
Spinach, boiled	½ cup	78 mg
Cashews, dry roasted	1 ounce	74 mg
Soymilk, plain or vanilla	1 cup	61 mg
Yogurt, nonfat	1 cup	47 mg
Tuna, canned in water	4 ounces	32 mg
Banana	1 medium	32 mg
Raisins	½ cup	23 mg
Broccoli, chopped and cooked	½ cup	12 mg

Magnesium is also available in multivitamin-mineral supplements and other dietary supplements. How well the magnesium in supplements is absorbed by the body varies depending on the form of magnesium. Forms of magnesium that are more easily absorbed are magnesium aspartate, magnesium citrate, magnesium lactate, and magnesium chloride. Some laxatives and products for treating heartburn and indigestion also include magnesium.

Recommended Dietary Allowances (RDAs) for Magnesium

LIFE STAGE GROUP	MILLIGRAMS PER DAY
Infants 0–6 months	30 mg*
Infants 7–12 months	75 mg*
Children 1–3 years	80 mg
Children 4–8 years	130 mg
Children 9–13 years	240 mg
Teen boys 14–18 years	410 mg
Teen girls 14–18 years	360 mg
Men 19–30 years	400 mg
Women 19–30 years	310 mg
Men 31+ years	420 mg
Women 31+ years	320 mg
Pregnant teens 14–18 years	400 mg
Pregnant women 19–30 years	350 mg
Pregnant women 31–50 years	360 mg
Breastfeeding teens 14–18 years	360 mg
Breastfeeding women 19–30 years	310 mg
Breastfeeding women 31–50 years	320 mg

*Adequate Intake (AI)

Magnesium Deficiency and Excess

Nutritional surveys show that most people in the United States get less than the recommended amounts of magnesium from food. Men over 70 and adolescent girls are the most likely to have low magnesium intakes. However, when magnesium from food and supplements are combined, the total intakes are usually above recommended amounts.

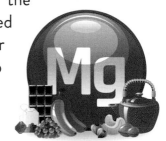

Loss of appetite, vomiting, nausea, fatigue, and weakness are early signs of magnesium deficiency. As the condition worsens, magnesium deficiency can cause numbness, tingling, muscle cramps, seizures, personality changes, and abnormal heart rhythms.

High intakes of magnesium from food are rarely a concern for healthy people since the kidneys eliminate excess amounts in urine. However, high doses of magnesium from dietary supplements can cause diarrhea, nausea, and abdominal cramps. Do not consume magnesium in dietary supplements in amounts above the upper limit unless instructed by a health care provider.

The risk of magnesium toxicity is greatest for people who absorb more magnesium than usual and those who cannot effectively excrete excess magnesium. This group includes older people and those with long-standing diabetes or kidney disease. People who have had intestinal surgery or who are taking medication to slow intestinal activity are also at higher risk of magnesium toxicity.

Magnesium and Health

A sufficient amount of magnesium is necessary to be sure the body is using calcium efficiently. Studies show that calcium supplements are not as effective in increasing bone density in people who are deficient in magnesium. In other words, calcium cannot correct bone loss if there is a magnesium deficiency. (The same is also true for vitamin D.)

Increasing intakes of magnesium from foods or dietary supplements may help older women improve their bone mineral density. Bone mineral density is important in reducing the risk of bone fractures and osteoporosis.

People whose diets include higher amounts of magnesium tend to have a lower risk of developing type 2 diabetes. Magnesium helps the body break down sugars and might help reduce the risk of insulin resistance—a condition that leads to diabetes.

Magnesium supplements might decrease blood pressure, but only by a small amount. Some studies show that people with high intakes of magnesium in their diets have a lower risk of some types of heart disease and stroke.

MANGANESE

Manganese is a mineral that helps ensure proper bone formation and connective-tissue growth. It activates many enzymes that regulate metabolism. It may also play a role as an antioxidant, as part of the enzyme superoxide dismutase.

Good sources of manganese include nuts, seeds, legumes, whole grains, tea, and leafy greens. Manganese is also available in dietary supplements. It is frequently included in supplements for osteoarthritis.

There is no RDA for manganese. However, safe and adequate intakes are shown in the table below. Taking more than the Tolerable Upper Intake Level (UL) can result in unwanted side effects. For most adults, the UL is 11 milligrams of manganese per day. People with liver disease and those with iron deficiency anemia should be especially careful not to get too much manganese.

ADEQUATE INTAKES (AIs) FOR MANGANESE

LIFE STAGE GROUP	MILLIGRAMS PER DAY
Infants 0–6 months	0.003 mg
Infants 7–12 months	0.6 mg
Children 1–3 years	1.2 mg
Children 4–8 years	1.5 mg
Boys 9–13 years	1.9 mg
Girls 9–13 years	1.6 mg
Teen boys 14–18 years	2.2 mg
Teen girls 14–18 years	1.6 mg
Men 19+ years	2.3 mg
Women 19+ years	1.8 mg
Pregnant teens and women	2.0 mg
Breastfeeding teens and women	2.6 mg

MELATONIN

Melatonin is a hormone produced by the pineal gland. It plays an important role in sleep. The production and release of melatonin is related to the time of day, rising at night and falling in the morning. Darkness signals the body to make melatonin while light blocks melatonin production.

Therapeutic Value of Melatonin

Research has shown that using melatonin may reduce jet lag symptoms and improve sleep after traveling across more than one time zone. Jet lag can cause disturbed sleep, daytime fatigue, indigestion, and a general feeling of discomfort. If you're trying to reset your body clock, take melatonin at local bedtime nightly until you have adapted to local time.

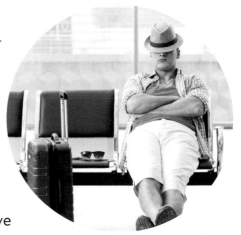

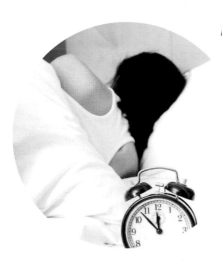

Melatonin has also been used as a tool to treat delayed sleep phase disorder (a disruption of the body's biological clock). Adolescents and adults with this disorder generally fall asleep well after midnight and have trouble waking up in the morning. When used in combination with reduced evening light and behavioral changes, melatonin supplements may help even out sleep cycles.

Some people who work afternoon to nighttime or nighttime to early morning hours are affected by shift work disorder. Melatonin supplements have been shown to improve daytime sleep quality and duration, but not nighttime alertness, in people with shift work disorder.

Melatonin supplements are also used for insomnia. A 2007 study of people ages 55 and up with insomnia found that prolonged-release melatonin significantly improved quality of sleep and morning alertness. Several studies of people with primary sleep disorders have found that melatonin slightly improved time to fall asleep, total sleep time, and overall sleep quality.

Sources of Melatonin

Melatonin is only made in the body; there are no food sources other than supplements. Melatonin is generally considered safe when taken short-term. Side effects are uncommon, but can include drowsiness, headache, dizziness, or nausea. Melatonin can interact with anticoagulants, anticonvulsants, birth control pills, immunosuppressants, and diabetes medications.

MILK THISTLE

Milk thistle (*Silybum marianum*) is native to central and western Europe and is grown elsewhere. The herb is primarily used for detoxifying and nourishing the liver.

The flavonoids in milk thistle appear to repair damaged liver cells, protect existing cells, and stimulate production of new liver cells. Milk thistle contains essential oils, tyramine, histamine, and silymarin. Milk thistle has antioxidant properties and is thought to counteract some of the detrimental effects of environmental toxins.

Milk thistle is available in capsules, tablets, powders, and extracts. In Europe, preparations made from silybin (found in milk thistle seeds) are given by intravenous infusion to victims of *Amanita* mushroom poisoning, which can be fatal.

Milk thistle and silymarin (the main component of milk thistle seeds) are generally considered safe when taken in recommended doses. Compounds in milk thistle may lower blood sugar levels in people with type 2 diabetes. People with diabetes should talk to a health care provider before using supplements.

MOLYBDENUM

This hard-to-pronounce mineral (muh LIB duh num) functions as part of the enzyme systems involved in carbohydrate, fat, and protein metabolism. Humans need only very small amounts of molybdenum, which are easily acquired through a healthy diet.

Good sources of molybdenum are liver, wheat germ, whole grains, nuts, and legumes. The molybdenum content of food varies according to what was in the soil from which it came.

RECOMMENDED DIETARY ALLOWANCES (RDAs) FOR MOLYBDENUM

LIFE STAGE GROUP	MICROGRAMS PER DAY
Infants 0–6 months	2 mcg*
Infants 7–12 months	3 mcg*
Children 1–3 years	17 mcg
Children 4–8 years	22 mcg
Children 9–13 years	34 mcg
Teens 14–18 years	43 mcg
Adults 19+ years	45 mcg
Pregnant and teens and women	50 mcg
Breastfeeding teens and women	50 mcg

*Adequate Intake (AI)

Molybdenum deficiency is very rare in humans, so supplements are rarely needed. The risk of molybdenum toxicity in humans from food sources is very low. The Tolerable Upper Intake Level (UL) for most adults is 2,000 micrograms (or 2 milligrams) per day. People who have a copper deficiency could be at increased risk of molybdenum toxicity.

NIACIN (VITAMIN B3)

Niacin, also known as nicotinic acid, is a form of vitamin B_3. The body needs niacin to convert food into energy, and to keep the nervous system, digestive tract, and skin healthy. Niacin is used to lower high blood pressure and cholesterol, and to treat niacin deficiency.

History

In the early part of the 18th century, a disease characterized by red, rough skin began to appear in Europe. Almost 200 years later, the disease was still a scourge—at least for people in the southern United States. The disease, called pellagra, was almost epidemic in the South by the early 1900s.

It was so common that many believed it was an infectious disease spread from person to person. Others thought eating spoiled corn caused it. Some even believed it was spread by a type of fly because outbreaks of the malady were more severe in the spring during flies' hatching season.

Few people believed that pellagra was a simple dietary deficiency, even though corn-based diets apparently made people susceptible to the disease. Dr. Joseph Goldberger (*right*) proved the link between diet and the disease by experimenting with the diets of children in a Mississippi orphanage who suffered from pellagra and 11 volunteers from a Mississippi prison farm. In both groups, when Goldberger added lean meat, milk, eggs, or yeast, their symptoms vanished.

This was in 1915, yet many physicians remained skeptical until 1937 when Conrad Elvehjem and his coworkers at the University of Wisconsin cured dogs with symptoms similar to pellagra by giving them nicotinic acid—a form of niacin. Soon doctors were using nicotinic acid to cure pellagra in humans.

Functions of Niacin

Niacin, a member of the vitamin B complex family, is a form of vitamin B_3. Another form of vitamin B_3 is niacinamide (also called nicotinamide). Niacinamide is formed from and converted to niacin in the body.

Like the other B vitamins thiamin and riboflavin, niacin acts as a coenzyme, assisting other substances in the conversion of proteins, carbohydrates, and fats into energy.

Sources of Niacin

Niacin is found in foods such as yeast, milk and other dairy products, eggs, lean meats, poultry, fish, legumes, nuts, and whole grains. Many breads and breakfast cereals are also fortified with niacin during manufacturing.

Niacin (nicotinic acid) is an ingredient in many multivitamin-mineral supplements, and also available as a standalone supplement.
Some niacin products are FDA-approved prescription drugs for treating abnormal levels of blood fats.

RECOMMENDED DIETARY ALLOWANCES (RDAs) FOR NIACIN

LIFE STAGE GROUP	MILLIGRAMS PER DAY
Infants 0–6 months	2 mg*
Infants 7–12 months	4 mg*
Children 1–3 years	6 mg
Children 4–8 years	8 mg
Children 9–13 years	12 mg
Teen boys 14–18 years	16 mg
Teen girls 14–18 years	14 mg
Men 19+ years	16 mg
Women 19+ years	14 mg
Pregnant teens and women	18 mg
Breastfeeding teens and women	17 mg

*Adequate Intake (AI)

Deficiency of Niacin

Pellagra is a disease of deficiency of niacin (vitamin B_3). It can result from an inability to absorb niacin or the amino acid tryptophan. The first symptoms of pellagra are weakness, loss of appetite, and some digestive disturbances. As the deficiency disease progresses, the skin becomes rough and red in areas exposed to sunlight, heat, or irritation. Later, open sores, diarrhea, dementia, and delirium may develop. Death results if the condition is left untreated.

This disease, now rarely seen in the United States, is still common in parts of the world where corn is the major cereal grain. Corn is deficient in tryptophan, and the niacin it contains is difficult to absorb. In many

Latin American countries, they combine cornmeal with the mineral lime when making tortillas; the alkalinity of the lime frees the niacin so that it can be absorbed.

Niacin Use and Misuse

Treatment for niacin deficiency commonly involves giving 25 to 50 milligrams (mg) of the vitamin daily. Larger doses of nicotinic acid, in amounts ranging from 500 milligrams (mg) to 3 grams (g) daily, have been used as a treatment option for low HDL "good" cholesterol and high LDL "bad" cholesterol and triglyceride levels.

Used in such large doses, however, nicotinic acid is no longer working as a vitamin, but as a drug, and side effects can occur. Large doses of niacin can cause an increased blood sugar (glucose) level, liver damage, peptic ulcers, and skin rashes.

Even normal doses of niacin can be associated with a condition called "flushing." This can result in feeling warmth, tingling, itching, and reddening of the face, neck, arms, or chest. The condition is uncomfortable, but not dangerous. To prevent flushing, do not drink hot beverages or alcohol at the same time as you take niacin. Niacinamide (nicotinamide) does not cause these side effects.

In addition, large doses of nicotinic acid can cause indigestion, peptic ulcers, injury to the liver, and an increased blood level of both uric acid and glucose. This can lead to misdiagnosis of diabetes or gout.

High doses of niacinamide do not typically cause any adverse reactions. But it's wise to always talk to your health care provider before starting any dietary supplement.

NICKEL

Nickel is a trace mineral present in tissues of the body. It is firmly attached to DNA and a protein that binds to it in the blood. While no clear biological function in humans has been identified, it may serve as a cofactor of metalloenzymes (enzymes containing tightly bound metal atoms) and may facilitate iron absorption.

OMEGA-3 FATTY ACIDS

Omega-3 fatty acids are found in foods and dietary supplements. There are three main omega-3s: alpha-linolenic acid (ALA), eicosapentaenoic acid (EPA), and docosahexaenoic acid (DHA). ALA is an essential fatty acid found mainly in plant oils such as flaxseed, soybean, and canola oils. DHA and EPA are found in fish and other seafood.

Sources of Omega-3s

Omega-3s are naturally present in some foods, including fish and other seafood (especially cold-water fatty fish), nuts and seeds, and plant and nut oils. Some foods, such as certain brands of eggs, yogurt, juices, milk, soy beverages, and infant formulas, are fortified with DHA and other omega-3s. Good food sources of omega-3s include salmon, mackerel, tuna, herring, sardines, flaxseeds, chia seeds, walnuts, flaxseed oil, soybean oil, canola oil, and fortified foods.

Omega-3s are also available in dietary supplements. Omega-3 supplements include fish oil, krill oil, cod liver oil, and algal oil (a vegetarian source that comes from algae). They come in a variety of doses and include various forms of omega-3s.

Recommended Intakes for Omega-3s

The table below shows the Adequate Intakes (AIs) for omega-3s in grams per day. For infants, the AIs apply to total omega-3s. For all other life stage groups, the AIs apply only to alpha-linolenic acid (ALA) because it is the only omega-3 that is essential.

ADEQUATE INTAKES (AIs) FOR OMEGA-3s

LIFE STAGE GROUP	GRAMS OF ALA PER DAY
Infants 0–12 months	0.5 g*
Children 1–3 years	0.7 g
Children 4–8 years	0.9 g
Boys 9–13 years	1.2 g
Girls 9–13 years	1.0 g
Teen boys 14–18 years	1.6 g
Teen girls 14–18 years	1.1 g
Men 19+ years	1.6 g
Women 19+ years	1.1 g
Pregnant teens and women	1.4 g
Breastfeeding teens and women	1.3 g

* As total omega-3s. All other values are for alpha-linolenic acid (ALA) alone.

PANTOTHENIC ACID (VITAMIN B5)

Pantothenic acid, also known as vitamin B_5, is an essential nutrient that is naturally present in some foods, added to other foods, and available as a dietary supplement. The body needs pantothenic acid to convert food into energy and to make red blood cells, certain hormones, and particular fats.

History

Unlike the discovery of other vitamins, when investigators discovered pantothenic acid in the 1930s, they weren't looking for the cause of a specific human disease. They were looking for a substance necessary for yeast to grow. Along the way, researchers noticed that diets lacking pantothenic acid caused certain disorders in animals, including a retarded growth rate, anemia, degenerated nerve tissue, decreased production of antibodies, ulcers, and malformed offspring.

Since many animal species proved to have a dietary requirement for pantothenic acid, scientists believed that people probably needed it too. Experiments in the 1950s tested how a diet without pantothenic acid affected humans. After three or four weeks on a highly purified diet that lacked only pantothenic acid, volunteers complained of weakness and an overall "unwell" feeling. One person had burning cramps.

A few volunteers received a diet not only deficient in pantothenic acid, but also containing a compound that specifically interfered with the vitamin. These people developed symptoms faster than those in the other group and complained of insomnia, depression, gastrointestinal problems, leg cramps, and a burning sensation in the hands and feet. In both groups, volunteers showed signs of reduced antibody production.

In everyone, symptoms disappeared after adding back pantothenic acid, proving that pantothenic acid was indeed an essential vitamin for humans.

Functions of Pantothenic Acid

Pantothenic acid, also called vitamin B_5, is a part of important biological compounds. One of these, called coenzyme A (CoA), is involved in the release of energy from carbohydrates, fats, and proteins and in the synthesis of certain compounds. The other, acyl carrier protein, participates in the synthesis of fats.

Sources of Pantothenic Acid

Almost all foods contain pantothenic acid in some amount. Pantothenic acid is also added to various foods, including some breakfast cereals and beverages. The best sources include an eclectic mix: eggs, beef, chicken, organ meats, legumes, peanuts, potatoes, avocado, broccoli, mushrooms, milk, whole-grain cereals, and yeast. Fresh vegetables are better sources than canned vegetables because the canning process reduces the amount of pantothenic acid available.

Pantothenic acid is available in dietary supplements containing only pantothenic acid, in combination with other B vitamins in B-complex supplements, and in some multivitamin-mineral supplements. Pantothenic acid in dietary supplements is often in the form of calcium pantothenate or pantethine.

Food Sources of Pantothenic Acid

FOOD	QUANTITY	MILLIGRAMS
Beef liver, boiled	3 ounces	8.3 mg
Shitake mushrooms, cut into pieces, cooked	½ cup	2.6 mg
Sunflower seeds	¼ cup	2.4 mg
Liverwurst spread	¼ cup	1.62 mg
Avocado, raw	½ avocado	1.0 mg
Milk, 2%	1 cup	0.9 mg
Mushrooms, white, stir fried, sliced	½ cup	0.8 mg
Egg, hard-boiled	1 large	0.7 mg
Ham, cured	3 ounces	0.66 mg
Broccoli, boiled	½ cup	0.5 mg
Peanuts, roasted in oil	¼ cup	0.5 mg
Cheddar cheese	1.5 ounces	0.2 mg

Adequate Intakes (AIs) for Pantothenic Acid

LIFE STAGE GROUP	MILLIGRAMS PER DAY
Infants 0–6 months	1.7 mg
Infants 7–12 months	1.8 mg
Children 1–3 years	2 mg
Children 4–8 years	3 mg
Children 9–13 years	4 mg
Teens 14–18 years	5 mg
Adults 19+ years	5 mg
Pregnant teens and women	6 mg
Breastfeeding teens and women	7 mg

Deficiency of Pantothenic Acid

Pantothenic acid deficiency is extremely rare in the United States. Most people get enough pantothenic acid by eating a varied diet. However, people with a rare inherited disorder called pantothenate kinase-associated neurodegeneration can't use pantothenic acid properly. Severe deficiency can cause numbness and burning of hands and feet, headache, extreme fatigue, irritability, restlessness, insomnia, stomach pain, heartburn, diarrhea, nausea, vomiting, and loss of appetite.

Pantothenic Acid Use and Misuse

Pantothenic acid is safe for most people. It is not known to interact with any medications. Massive doses of pantothenic acid (as much as 10 to 20 grams a day) have been reported to cause mild diarrhea in some people, but serious toxicity is not known to occur.

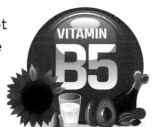

PARA-AMINOBENZOIC ACID

Para-aminobenzoic acid (PABA) is part of the B vitamin folate and, therefore, isn't considered a separate vitamin. PABA is best known for its use in sunscreens. When applied to skin, PABA can help protect against sunburn. Taken orally, however, PABA does not have the same protective effect. Large doses taken over extended periods can cause nausea and vomiting. Oral use is not recommended.

PHOSPHORUS

Phosphorus is a mineral that is vital for strong bones and teeth. Phosphorus also plays an important role in energy storage and release. It's found in DNA (deoxyribonucleic acid) and RNA (ribonucleic acid), the genetic materials that serve as the blueprints for the formation of new cells. Phosphorus is necessary for normal milk secretion and a variety of metabolic reactions as well.

Sources of Phosphorus

Good sources of phosphorus are also good sources of protein—for example, such foods as milk and other dairy products, eggs, meat, fish, poultry, nuts, and whole grains are good sources of both. Fruits and vegetables contain only small amounts of phosphorus. Phosphorus is added to many processed foods. Even sodas and food additives supply some phosphorous. As a result, most Americans get plenty of phosphorus from their diet.

FOOD SOURCES OF PHOSPHORUS

FOOD	QUANTITY	MILLIGRAMS
Sardines, Atlantic, canned	3 ounces	412 mg
Kidney beans, canned	1 cup	254 mg
Milk, skim	1 cup	247 mg
Almonds, roasted	1/4 cup	205 mg
Tuna, canned in water	3 ounces	156 mg

Recommended Dietary Allowances (RDAs) for Phosphorus

LIFE STAGE GROUP	MILLIGRAMS
Infants 0–6 months	100 mg*
Infants 7–12 months	275 mg*
Children 1–3 years	460 mg
Children 4–8 years	500 mg
Children 9–13 years	1,250 mg
Teens 14–18 years	1,250 mg
Adults 19+ years	700 mg
Pregnant and breastfeeding teens under 18	1,250 mg
Pregnant and breastfeeding women over 18	700 mg

*Adequate Intake (AI)

Phosphorus Deficiency and Excess

A true phosphorus deficiency is rare in the United States because the mineral is so readily available in the food supply. In fact, Americans consume as much as four times their recommended dietary allowance. American diets are heavy in high-protein foods (such as meat, fish, or poultry), carbonated beverages, and ready-to-eat convenience foods—all of which increase the body's supply of phosphorus. However, phosphorus deficiency has been reported in some infants fed cow's milk and in some people taking large amounts of antacids.

Excessively high levels of phosphorus in the blood typically only occur in people with severe kidney disease or severe dysfunction of their calcium regulation.

PHYTOCHEMICALS

Phytochemicals, also called phytonutrients, are natural substances found in plants that help protect the plant from disease. In humans, phytonutrients have numerous health-promoting properties; they function as antioxidants to help rid the body of toxins and prevent inflammation.

POTASSIUM

Potassium is a mineral that the body needs for cells, nerves, and muscles to function properly. Potassium plays an important role in maintaining water balance and acid-base balance. Its presence is crucial in the transmission of nerve impulses from nerves to muscles. It also acts as a catalyst in carbohydrate and protein metabolism.

Sources of Potassium

While almost all whole foods contain some potassium, particularly good sources include apricots, prunes, legumes, squash, potatoes, milk, tomatoes, bananas, oranges, and meat. Fruits and vegetables reign supreme in the potassium-supply category. Processed foods, on the other hand, lose much of their potassium.

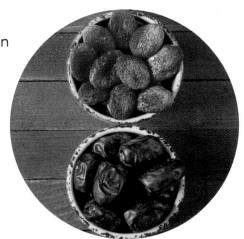

Potassium combined with chloride is effective at restoring potassium losses from the body and can satisfy a taste for table salt. In fact, many salt substitutes are compounds of potassium chloride. People with kidney disease, however, should avoid them.

Potassium is included in many multivitamin-mineral supplements and in supplements that contain only potassium. In dietary supplements, potassium is often in the form of potassium chloride. However, many other forms of potassium, including potassium citrate, phosphate, aspartate, bicarbonate, and gluconate, are also used in supplements.

FOOD SOURCES OF POTASSIUM

FOOD	QUANTITY	MILLIGRAMS
Apricots, dried	½ cup	1,101 mg
Lentils, cooked	1 cup	731 mg
Prunes, dried	½ cup	699 mg
Acorn squash, mashed	1 cup	644 mg
Kidney beans, canned	1 cup	607 mg
Orange juice	1 cup	496 mg
Banana	1 medium	422 mg
Milk, 1%	1 cup	366 mg
Spinach, raw	2 cups	334 mg

ADEQUATE INTAKES (AIs) FOR POTASSIUM

LIFE STAGE GROUP	MILLIGRAMS PER DAY
Infants 0–6 months	400 mg
Infants 7–12 months	700 mg
Children 1–3 years	3,000 mg
Children 4–8 years	3,800 mg
Children 9–13 years	4,500 mg
Teens 14–18 years	4,700 mg
Adults 19+ years	4,700 mg
Pregnant teens and women	4,700 mg
Breastfeeding teens and women	5,100 mg

Potassium Deficiency and Excess

Having too much or too little potassium in the body can cause serious health problems. A low level of potassium is called hypokalemia. A high level of potassium in the blood is called hyperkalemia.

Dietary surveys consistently show that most people in the United States consume much less potassium than recommended, which is why the *2015-2020 Dietary Guidelines for Americans* identifies potassium as a nutrient of public health concern. Not getting enough potassium can increase blood pressure, deplete calcium in bones, and increase the risk of kidney stones.

Hypokalemia can be caused by certain kidney or adrenal gland disorders, prolonged vomiting and diarrhea, laxative abuse, use of diuretics, excessive sweating, and dialysis. Symptoms of hypokalemia include constipation, tiredness, muscle weakness, increased urination, decreased brain function, high blood sugar levels, muscle paralysis, difficulty breathing, and irregular heartbeat.

Too much potassium in the blood is known as hyperkalemia. It can cause abnormal and dangerous heart rhythms. Some common causes include the types of heart medications called angiotensin converting enzyme (ACE) inhibitors and angiotensin 2 receptor blockers (ARBs), poor kidney function, potassium-sparing diuretics (water pills), and severe infection.

PROBIOTICS

Probiotics are live bacteria and other microorganisms that are good for you. The most common microorganisms in probiotics are bacteria that belong to two broad groups called *Lactobacillus* and *Bifidobacterium*.

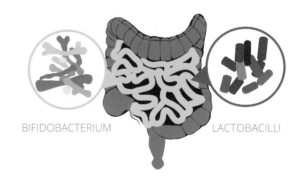

BIFIDOBACTERIUM

LACTOBACILLI

DIGESTIVE SYSTEMS

Probiotics are often promoted for digestive health. Preliminary evidence shows that some probiotics may be helpful in preventing diarrhea caused by infections and antibiotics and in improving irritable bowel syndrome symptoms, but further study is needed.

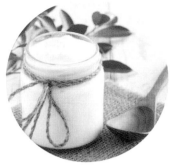

Probiotics are found in dietary supplements and foods such as yogurt. To get the probiotic benefits in yogurt, be sure to check the label on the carton for the National Yogurt Association's "Live & Active Cultures" (LAC) seal. This seal identifies products that contain a significant amount of live and active cultures.

RED CLOVER

Like beans and peas, red clover (*Trifolium pratense*) belongs to the legume plant family. Red clover contains substances called isoflavones. Isoflavones are phytoestrogens—compounds similar to the female hormone estrogen. Red clover also contains the blood-thinning substance coumarin.

Historically, red clover has been used to treat everything from asthma, coughs, and respiratory system congestion to cancer and gout.
Today, people use isoflavone extracts from red clover as dietary supplements for menopausal symptoms, high cholesterol, or osteoporosis. The flowering tops of the red clover plant are often used to prepare extracts available in tablets, capsules, teas, and liquid forms.

The raw greens of this plant are very nutritious, but like other members of the legume family, they are somewhat difficult to digest. The leaves are best enjoyed dried and in the tea form to get the nutrients and constituents without the side effects of gas and bloating common to eating legumes.

When to Avoid Red Clover

Those with abnormally low platelet counts, those using anticoagulant drugs, and those with clotting defects should avoid red clover. Do not consume red clover before surgery or childbirth, as it may impair the ability of the blood to clot. Red clover is believed to promote the growth of uterine fibroids in sheep, but whether this is true for humans is unknown. There is also some concern that red clover may stimulate cancers that are fed by estrogen, such as some breast and uterine cancers. Until more is known, it may be best for patients with hormonally influenced cancers or uterine fibroids to avoid red clover.

RESVERATROL

Resveratrol is an antioxidant-like compound found in red wine, red grape skins, purple grape juice, and mulberries.

Resveratrol appears to help control blood sugar levels and improve how well insulin works in people with type 2 diabetes. Some research shows that resveratrol might be linked to a lower risk of inflammation and blood clotting, which can lead to heart disease. But other studies found no benefits from resveratrol in preventing heart disease.

RETINOIDS

Retinoids are a class of compounds related to vitamin A. Some retinoids include retinol, retinal, and retinoic acid. Synthetic retinoids are sometimes used for skin disorders. For more information, see the full vitamin A profile on page 156.

RETINOL (VITAMIN A)

Retinol, also called preformed vitamin A, is a form of vitamin A found in foods that come from animals. Retinol can be used by the body to make retinal and retinoic acid (other forms of vitamin A). See the full vitamin A profile on page 156.

RIBOFLAVIN (VITAMIN B2)

Riboflavin (also called vitamin B_2) is important for cell growth, development, and function. It also helps turn food into energy.

History

Most nutritionists in the 1920s believed that there were only two unidentified essential nutrients—a fat-soluble A and a water-soluble B. Soon, however, they found there was a second water-soluble B compound waiting to be identified.

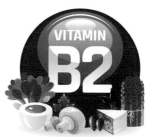

During the course of their work, nutritionists gradually isolated growth-producing substances from liver, eggs, milk, and grass. All of the substances were yellow. In 1933, L.E. Booher reported that she had also obtained a yellow growth-promoting substance from milk whey. In addition, she observed that the darker the color of the substance, the greater its potency. Booher's observation led nutritionists to discover that all the yellow growth-producing substances in foods were one and the same—riboflavin.

While nutritionists zeroed in on the yellow substance in food, biochemists studied a yellow enzyme found to be essential for the body's energy needs. Biochemists were eventually able to separate the enzyme into two parts: a colorless protein and a yellow organic compound that turned out to be the riboflavin itself.

Functions of Riboflavin

Riboflavin acts as a coenzyme—the non-protein, active portion of an enzyme—by helping to metabolize carbohydrates, fats, and proteins to provide the body with energy. Riboflavin doesn't act alone, however; it works in concert with its B-complex relatives. Riboflavin also plays a role in the metabolism of other vitamins.

Sources of Riboflavin

Riboflavin is found naturally in some foods and is added to many fortified foods. Eggs, organ meats, lean meats, and milk are particularly rich in riboflavin. Green vegetables such as asparagus, broccoli, and spinach also provide some riboflavin. Riboflavin is added to many fortified cereals, breads, and grain products. The daily value (DV) for riboflavin, which was established by the FDA, is 1.7 milligrams for adults and children age 4 and older.

Protect Your Riboflavin

Milk in plastic jugs is more susceptible to loss of riboflavin and vitamin A than milk in paperboard cartons. That's because light, even the fluorescent light in supermarkets, destroys these two light-sensitive nutrients.

Riboflavin is available in many dietary supplements. You can find riboflavin in multivitamin-mineral supplements, in B-complex dietary supplements, and in riboflavin-only supplements. Some supplements have much more than the recommended amounts of riboflavin, but the body can't absorb more than about 27 milligrams at a time.

FOOD SOURCES OF RIBOFLAVIN

FOOD	QUANTITY	MILLIGRAMS
Beef liver, pan fried	3 ounces	2.9 mg
Yogurt, plain, fat free	1 cup	0.6 mg
Milk, 2%	1 cup	0.5 mg
Swiss cheese	3 ounces	0.3 mg
Egg, whole, scrambled	1 large	0.2 mg
Spinach, raw	1 cup	0.1 mg

RECOMMENDED DIETARY ALLOWANCES (RDAs) FOR RIBOFLAVIN

LIFE STAGE GROUP	MILLIGRAMS PER DAY
Infants 0–6 months	0.3 mg*
Infants 7–12 months	0.4 mg*
Children 1–3 years	0.5 mg
Children 4–8 years	0.6 mg
Children 9–13 years	0.9 mg
Teen boys 14–18 years	1.3 mg
Teen girls 14–18 years	1.0 mg
Men 19+ years	1.3 mg
Women 19+ years	1.1 mg
Pregnant teens and women	1.4 mg
Breastfeeding teens and women	1.6 mg

*Adequate Intake (AI)

Deficiency of Riboflavin

Most people in the United States get enough riboflavin from the foods they eat and deficiencies are extremely rare. Riboflavin deficiency can cause skin disorders, sores at the corners of the mouth, swollen and cracked lips, hair loss, sore throat, liver disorders, and problems with the reproductive and nervous systems. Anemia and cataracts can develop if riboflavin deficiency is severe and prolonged.

Riboflavin Use and Misuse

Riboflavin has not been shown to cause any harm, and is not known to interact with any medications. However, it's important to tell your healthcare providers about any dietary supplements and prescription or over-the-counter medicines you take.

SAW PALMETTO

Saw palmetto is a small palm tree native to the southeastern United States. Extracts of its fruit are used in tablets or capsules. Saw palmetto has also been used as ground, dried, or whole berries, a liquid extract, or a tea. Saw palmetto is used for urinary symptoms associated with an enlarged prostate gland and many other conditions, including decreased sex drive, hair loss, and chronic pelvic pain.

SELENIUM

Selenium is a mineral important for reproduction, thyroid gland function, DNA production, and protecting the body from free radical damage and infection.

Functions of Selenium

Selenium functions as an antioxidant as part of the enzyme glutathione peroxidase. It helps prevent cell damage from free radicals that form when oxygen attacks, or oxidizes, fats and other compounds. Severe deficiency of selenium affects heart function, but a deficiency is hard to detect because vitamin E can substitute for selenium in some of its functions, thus masking the classic symptoms.

Sources of Selenium

Selenium is naturally present in many foods. The amount of selenium in plant foods depends on the selenium content of the soil in which they were grown. For animal products, the amount depends on the selenium content of the foods the animals ate.

A super source of selenium is the Brazil nut, with 68–91 micrograms (mcg) per nut. Seafood and organ meats are also rich in selenium. Other food sources include poultry, eggs, dairy products, breads, cereals, and other grain products. The daily value (DV) for selenium is 70 micrograms for adults and children over age 4.

Selenium is also available in many multivitamin-mineral supplements and in standalone supplements. The selenium in supplements often comes in the forms of selenomethionine or sodium selenite.

FOOD SOURCES OF SELENIUM

FOOD	QUANTITY	MICROGRAMS
Brazil nuts	1 ounce	544 mcg
Shrimp, canned	3 ounces	40 mcg
Turkey, boneless, roasted	3 ounces	31 mcg
Beef liver, pan fried	3 ounces	28 mcg
Egg, hard-boiled	1 large	15 mcg
Milk, 1%	1 cup	8 mcg

RECOMMENDED DIETARY ALLOWANCES (RDAs) FOR SELENIUM

LIFE STAGE GROUP	MICROGRAMS PER DAY
Infants 0–6 months	15 mcg*
Infants 7–12 months	20 mcg*
Children 1–3 years	20 mcg
Children 4–8 years	30 mcg
Children 9–13 years	40 mcg
Teens 14–18 years	55 mcg
Adults 19+ years	55 mcg
Pregnant teens and women	60 mcg
Breastfeeding teens and women	70 mcg

*Adequate Intake (AI)

Selenium Deficiency and Excess

Most Americans consume adequate amounts of selenium, so deficiency is extremely rare in the United States. Selenium deficiency can cause a type of heart disease called Keshan disease and male infertility. It might also cause Kashin-Beck disease, a type of osteoarthritis that produces pain, swelling, and loss of motion in the joints.

Too much selenium can be toxic because this mineral can substitute for sulfur in the proteins of some important enzymes, altering their functions. So if you take selenium supplements, they should contain no more than the RDA. The Tolerable Upper Intake Levels (ULs) for selenium are shown below. Selenium taken as seleno-amino acid is much less toxic because the selenium substitution has already been made.

Signs and symptoms of chronically high selenium intakes include hair and nail loss or brittleness, nausea, diarrhea, skin rashes, discolored teeth, fatigue, irritability, and nervous system abnormalities. Extremely high intakes of selenium can cause difficulty breathing, tremors, kidney failure, heart attacks, and heart failure.

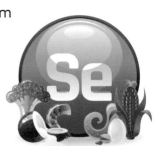

TOLERABLE UPPER INTAKE LEVELS (ULs) FOR SELENIUM*

LIFE STAGE GROUP	MICROGRAMS PER DAY
Infants 0–6 months	45 mcg
Infants 7–12 months	60 mcg
Children 1–3 years	90 mcg
Children 4–8 years	150 mcg
Children 9–13 years	280 mcg
Teens 14–18 years	400 mcg
Adults 19+ years	400 mcg
Pregnant teens and women	400 mcg
Breastfeeding teens and women	400 mcg

*Breast milk, formula, and food should be the only sources of selenium for infants.

SLIPPERY ELM

Slippery elm is a tree whose inner bark is used for various purposes, including sore throat. Some commercial lozenges for cough and sore throat contain slippery elm. Added to water, the powdered bark becomes a soothing mucilage. The mucilage moistens and soothes while the herb's tannins are astringent, making slippery elm ideal to reduce inflammation and swelling, and heal damaged tissues. Mucilage is the most abundant constituent of slippery elm bark, but the tree also contains starch, sugar, calcium, iodine, bromine, amino acids, and traces of manganese and zinc. Many people eat slippery elm to soothe and nourish the body. Slippery elm helps heal internal mucosal tissues, such as the stomach, vagina, and esophagus. It is often recommended as a restorative herb for people who suffer from prolonged flu, stomach upset, chronic indigestion, and resulting malnutrition. You can use slippery elm to soothe ulcers and stomach inflammation, irritated intestines, vaginal inflammation, sore throat, coughs, and a hoarse voice.

SODIUM

Sodium plays a critical role in regulating water balance in the body. It's also important for regulating acid-base balance, transmitting nerve impulses, maintaining muscle activity and cell membrane function, and absorbing and transporting certain nutrients. Sodium is also a part of body fluids such as sweat and tears.

Recommended Intakes for Sodium

On average, Americans consume more than 3,400 milligrams of sodium per day. This far exceeds what the body actually needs to function properly. The *2015–2020 Dietary Guidelines for Americans* recommends limiting sodium to less than 2,300 milligrams per day. This is an upper limit, not a recommended daily allowance. Certain groups, including adults with prehypertension and hypertension, should limit intake to 1,500 milligrams per day. Sodium sensitive people should also further limit sodium intake. Sodium sensitive people retain sodium more easily, leading to fluid retention and increased blood pressure (hypertension).

Sources of Sodium

The majority of sodium in the typical American diet comes from processed and prepared foods. Processed foods include bread, crackers, breakfast cereals, pizza, microwavable dinners, canned vegetables, soups, sauces, deli meat, cheese, fast foods, and prepared dinners such as pasta, meat, and egg dishes.

Sodium is naturally present in some foods, including vegetables, dairy products, meat, and shellfish. Celery, carrots, artichokes, beets, eggs, and milk are naturally high in sodium.

Another source of sodium is the salt used in cooking or at the table. Common table salt consists of about 40 percent sodium and 60 percent chloride.

Sodium Deficiency and Excess

Because the body has a large sodium reserve and, under normal circumstances, people eat plenty of sodium-containing foods, a deficiency is not likely. However, salt depletion can temporarily occur through profuse sweating if you exercise strenuously for a prolonged time in warm weather or hot climates. Even in this situation, salt that's lost is easily replaced.

Excessive intake of sodium is a much more common problem than deficiency. Consuming too much sodium puts you at risk for developing serious medical conditions like high blood pressure (hypertension), heart disease, and stroke.

ST. JOHN'S WORT

St. John's wort (*Hypericum perforatum*) is a plant that has been used for centuries for mental health conditions. Today, people use St. John's wort as a dietary supplement for depression, menopausal symptoms, attention-deficit hyperactivity disorder (ADHD), and obsessive-compulsive disorder. It is also used topically for wound healing.

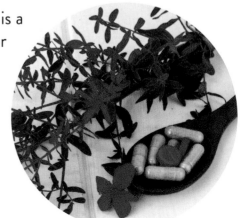

The plant, especially its tiny yellow flowers, is high in hypericin and other flavonoid compounds. If you crush a flower bud between your fingers, you will release a burgundy red juice—evidence of the flavonoid hypericin. St. John's wort oils and tinctures should display this beautiful red coloring, which indicates the presence of the desired flavonoids. Bioflavonoids, in general, serve to reduce vascular fragility and inflammation. Since flavonoids improve venous wall integrity, St. John's wort is useful in treating swollen veins.

Uses of St. John's Wort

St. John's wort is reported to relieve anxiety and tension and to act as an antidepressant. It was once thought that hypericin interferes with the body's production of a depression-related chemical called monoamine oxidase (MAO), but recent research has shed doubt on this claim. Though no one is yet certain how the herb works, studies have shown St. John's wort to act as a mood elevator in AIDS patients and in depressed subjects in general. However, St. John's wort is not consistently effective for depression. St. John's wort can also make some antidepressants less effective. Combining St. John's wort supplements and certain antidepressants can lead to a potentially life-threatening increase in the body's levels of serotonin.

St. John's wort preparations may be ingested for internal bruising and inflammation or following a traumatic injury to external muscles and skin. The oil is also useful when applied to wounds and bruises or rubbed onto strains, sprains, or varicose veins. When rubbed onto the belly and breasts during pregnancy, the oil may also help prevent stretch marks.

Topical application is also useful to treat hemorrhoids and aching, swollen veins that can occur during pregnancy.

St. John's wort is useful for pelvic pain and cramping. According to the 1983 *British Herbal Pharmacopoeia*, St. John's wort is specifically indicated for "menopausal neuroses": Many women who experience anxiety, depression, and other emotional disturbances during menopause may benefit from this herb's use. The National Cancer Institute has conducted several studies showing that St. John's wort has potential as a cancer-fighting drug. One study showed that mice injected with the feline leukemia virus were able to fight off the infection after just a single dose of St. John's wort.

Risks of St. John's Wort

St. John's wort can interact with a variety of medicines in dangerous, sometimes life-threatening ways. It can also weaken the effects of many medicines, including antidepressants; birth control pills; cyclosporine, which prevents the body from rejecting transplanted organs; digoxin, a heart medication; some HIV drugs, including indinavir; some cancer medications, including irinotecan; and warfarin, an anticoagulant. It is especially important to tell all of your health care providers if you plan to take St. John's wort because the herb interacts with so many medicines.

SULFUR

Sulfur is found throughout the body, especially in the skin, hair, and nails. The mineral aids in the storage and release of energy. It's a component of the genetic material of cells, and it helps promote enzyme reactions and blood clotting. Sulfur is part of two B vitamins—biotin and thiamin. Sulfur also combines with certain toxic materials so they can then be excreted safely from the body through the urine.

Although there is no RDA for sulfur, it's not because it plays an unimportant role. When protein intake is adequate, sulfur intake is adequate as well. That's because sulfur-containing amino acids (the building blocks of protein) supply the body with the amount of sulfur it needs. However, getting adequate amounts of sulfur from other sources preserves these amino acids for their other vital functions.

A wide variety of foods contain sulfur. Cheese, eggs, fish, poultry, grains, nuts, and dried peas and beans are all rich sources.

THIAMIN (VITAMIN B1)

Thiamin (also known as vitamin B_1) is important for energy metabolism, cell and muscle function, and nervous system health. The discovery of thiamin was the key that unlocked the mystery of a disease called beriberi.

History

Beriberi, a debilitating, often fatal ailment, wasn't a serious health problem among the rice-eating peoples of Asia until the end of the 19th century when mills began to polish rice. This process removes the outer brown layers of the grain, leaving behind smooth, white kernels. Rice stripped of this outer layer of bran loses much of its thiamin.

Not surprisingly, soon after this refining practice began, the incidence of beriberi rose to epidemic levels in Asia. A similar situation occurred in countries where wheat was a dietary staple when refined white flour began to replace whole-wheat flour. The increased prevalence of beriberi spurred efforts to find its cause and cure. Still, the search took almost 50 years and did not end until thiamin was discovered.

A medical officer in the Japanese navy named Kanehiro Takaki (right) was the first to suspect the relationship between diet and beriberi. In the 1880s, Takaki sought the root of this disease, which afflicted large numbers of Japanese sailors on long voyages—a situation reminiscent of scurvy. To test his belief that diet was at fault, Takaki added meat and milk to the rice diet of the sailors. Only a few men came down with the malady—those who refused to eat the milk and meat.

Further evidence came from the Indonesian island of Java, where the Dutch physician Christiaan Eijkman found that chickens fed polished rice exhibited symptoms similar to those of beriberi. When he fed the chickens unpolished rice, the symptoms soon disappeared. Eijkman then tried the same experiment on people and confirmed that unpolished rice could prevent and cure beriberi.

Still, it wasn't until 1910 that researchers began searching in earnest for the mystery substance in unpolished rice. Chemist Robert R. Williams analyzed liquid extracted from rice polishings, painstakingly testing each substance from it for its effect on polyneuritis, the chicken disease similar to beriberi. In 1934, Williams isolated the substance that would solve the beriberi riddle—the vitamin thiamin.

Functions of Thiamin

Like other B-complex vitamins, thiamin acts as a biological catalyst, or coenzyme. As a coenzyme, thiamin participates in the long chain of reactions that provides energy for the body and heat. Thiamin helps the body manufacture fats and metabolize protein. It's also needed for normal functioning of the nervous system.

Sources of Thiamin

Thiamin is naturally found in some foods and added to other food products. Enriched breads and cereals, meat (especially pork), fish, legumes, seeds, nuts, and whole grains are good sources of thiamin. Most other foods, fruits, and dairy products contain only small amounts

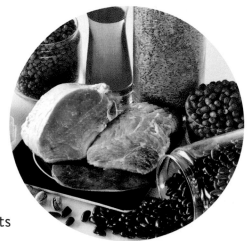

of thiamin. The daily value (DV) for thiamin is 1.5 milligrams for adults and children over age 4.

Heating foods containing thiamin at high temperatures can reduce their thiamin content. As a water-soluble vitamin, thiamin also tends to leach out of food into the cooking water. In order to preserve thiamin, it's best to cook food over low temperatures in small amounts of water for short periods. Steaming and microwaving can help minimize losses of thiamin and preserve the natural flavors of the foods. Sulfites, used as preservatives, also destroy thiamin. Your best bet for preserving a food's thiamin content is to use additives sparingly and keep the cooking time short.

Thiamin is available in multivitamin-mineral supplements, in B-complex supplements, and in standalone thiamin supplements. Common forms of thiamin in dietary supplements are thiamin mononitrate and thiamin hydrochloride. Some supplements use a synthetic form of thiamin called benfotiamine.

FOOD SOURCES OF THIAMIN

FOOD	QUANTITY	MILLIGRAMS
Breakfast cereal fortified with 100% DV of thiamin	1 serving	1.5 mg
Pork chop, bone-in, broiled	3 ounces	0.4 mg
Black beans, boiled	½ cup	0.4 mg
Mussels, blue, cooked, moist heat	3 ounces	0.3 mg
Tuna, Bluefin, cooked, dry heat	3 ounces	0.2 mg
Acorn squash, cubed, baked	½ cup	0.2 mg
Sunflower seeds, toasted	1 ounce	0.1 mg

RECOMMENDED DIETARY ALLOWANCES (RDAs) FOR THIAMIN

LIFE STAGE GROUP	MILLIGRAMS PER DAY
Infants 0–6 months	0.2 mg*
Infants 7–12 months	0.3 mg*
Children 1–3 years	0.5 mg
Children 4–8 years	0.6 mg
Children 9–13 years	0.9 mg
Teen boys 14–18 years	1.2 mg
Teen girls 14–18 years	1.0 mg
Men 19+ years	1.2 mg
Women 19+ years	1.1 mg
Pregnant teens and women	1.4 mg
Breastfeeding teens and women	1.4 mg

*Adequate Intake (AI)

Deficiency of Thiamin

A thiamin deficiency can develop if the body eliminates too much or absorbs too little thiamin, or if there's insufficient thiamin in the diet. Diets deficient in thiamin are often deficient in other B vitamins as well.

Signs and symptoms of thiamin deficiency include weight loss, loss of appetite, confusion, memory loss, muscle weakness, and heart problems. Severe thiamin deficiency leads to beriberi disease with the added symptoms of tingling and numbness in the feet and hands, muscle loss, and poor reflexes.

Severe thiamin deficiency (beriberi disease) seldom occurs today in the United States. However, a more common example of thiamin deficiency in the U.S. is Wernicke-Korsakoff syndrome, which mostly affects people with alcohol dependence. It causes tingling and numbness in the hands and feet, severe memory loss, disorientation, and confusion.

Thiamin and Health

Thiamin supplements are used for a variety of potential health benefits. In addition to helping prevent and treat thiamin deficiency, thiamin has been shown to help correct certain inherited metabolic disorders. Thiamin also seems to help decrease the risk and symptoms of the brain disorder Wernicke-Korsakoff syndrome, which is often seen in alcoholics.

TURMERIC

Turmeric is a spice that comes from the turmeric plant, which is grown in India and other parts of Asia. But this bright yellow spice isn't just for curries and teas. Turmeric is also used as a dietary supplement. People take turmeric supplements for inflammation; arthritis; skin, liver, and gallbladder problems; stomach pain; heartburn; and cancer. Researchers are studying curcumin, the active chemical in turmeric, for its possible health benefits.

UVA URSI

Uva ursi is used primarily to treat urinary problems, including bladder infections. The herb is disinfecting and promotes urine flow. Uva ursi is particularly recommended to treat illnesses caused by *Escherichia coli (E. coli)*, a bacterium that lives in the intestines and commonly causes bladder and kidney infections. For kidney infections or kidney stones, take the herb under the care of a naturopathic or other trained physician.

VALERIAN

Valerian is a flowering plant used as a dietary supplement for insomnia, tension, and nervousness. Despite what some people have come to believe, valerian is not the source of the drug Valium. However, valerian is a common ingredient in products promoted as mild sedatives and sleep aids for nervous tension and insomnia. Valerian also has an antispasmodic action and is used for cramps, muscle pain, and muscle tension.

Valerian is useful in simple cases of stress, anxiety, and nervous tension, as well as more severe cases of hysteria, nervous twitching, hyperactivity, chorea (involuntary jerky movements), heart palpitations, and tension headaches. Valerian is generally considered safe for healthy adults to use for short periods of time, but there is no information available on the long-term safety.

VITAMIN A

In the case of vitamin A, the eyes have it. The essential nutrient vitamin A plays a vital role in vision. Vitamin A is also important for reproduction, immunity, and cell development. In addition, vitamin A helps heart, lungs, kidneys, and other organs function properly.

There are two different types of vitamin A—preformed vitamin A (retinol) and provitamin A carotenoids. Retinol (or preformed vitamin A) is found in foods from animal sources. Provitamin A carotenoids are found in fruits, vegetables, and other plant-based products.

History

As indicated by its position at the head of the vitamin alphabet, vitamin A was the first vitamin discovered. In the early 1900s, researchers recognized that a certain substance in animal fats and fish oils was necessary for the growth of young animals. Scientists originally called the substance fat-soluble A to signify its presence in animal fats. Later, they renamed it vitamin A.

Functions of Vitamin A

The most clearly defined role of vitamin A is the part it plays in vision, especially the ability to see in the dark. Vitamin A deficiency is a major cause of blindness in the world.

Vitamin A is also important for normal growth and reproduction—especially proper development of bones and teeth. Animal studies show that vitamin A is essential for normal sperm formation, for growth of a healthy fetus, and perhaps for the synthesis of steroid hormones.

Another important, but misunderstood, role of vitamin A involves preserving healthy skin—inside and out. Taking extra vitamin A won't make your sagging skin suddenly beautiful, but a deficiency of it will cause skin problems. Furthermore, an adequate vitamin A intake ensures healthy mucous membranes of the gastrointestinal and respiratory tracts. In this way, vitamin A helps the body resist infection.

Sources of Vitamin A

Both plant and animal foods have vitamin A activity. Retinol, also called preformed vitamin A, is the natural form found in animals. Carotenoids, found in plants, are compounds that the body can convert to vitamin A. These precursors to vitamin A are sometimes called provitamin A. Bright-orange beta-carotene is the most important carotenoid for adequate vitamin A intake because it yields more vitamin A than alpha- or gamma-carotene.

Some carotenoids, such as lycopene, do not convert to vitamin A at all. Lycopene, the orange-red pigment found in tomatoes and watermelon, is still of value, however, because it's an antioxidant even more potent than beta-carotene. (See Chapter 4 for more on antioxidants.)

Liver is one of the best food sources of vitamin A. However, many experts recommend limiting consumption to once or twice a month because of the toxic substances it can contain. Environmental pollutants tend to congregate in an animal's liver. Egg yolk, cheese, whole milk, butter, fortified skim milk, and margarine are also good sources of vitamin A. Be careful, though, as all these foods—except fortified skim milk—are also high in total fat and saturated fat, and all except margarine are high in cholesterol.

Because of the high fat and cholesterol content of these foods, as well as the potential for overdosing, it is recommended that you do not look to these sources to fulfill your need for vitamin A. Instead, rely on the provitamin plant forms of carotenoids, which do not accumulate in your liver.

Orange and yellow fruits and vegetables have high vitamin A activity because of the carotenoids they contain. Generally, the deeper the color of the fruit or vegetable, the higher the concentration of carotenoids it has. Carrots, for example, are especially good sources of beta-carotene and, therefore, are high in vitamin A value. Green vegetables, such as spinach, asparagus, and broccoli, also contain large amounts of carotenoids, but their intense green pigment, courtesy of chlorophyll, masks the telltale orange-yellow color.

Most other carotenoids, such as alpha- and gamma-carotene, plus cryptoxanthin and beta-zeacarotene have less vitamin A activity than beta-carotene, but offer ample cancer prevention. Some carotenoids, such as lycopene, zeaxanthin, lutein, capsanthin, and canthaxanthin are not converted into vitamin A in the body. But again, they are powerful cancer fighters, prevalent in both fruits and vegetables.

In addition to food sources, vitamin A is also available in dietary supplements. The vitamin A in supplements is usually in the form of retinyl acetate or retinyl palmitate (preformed vitamin A), beta-carotene (provitamin A), or a combination of preformed and provitamin A. Most multivitamin-mineral supplements contain vitamin A. You can also buy standalone vitamin A supplements.

Recommended Intakes for Vitamin A

The RDAs for vitamin A are given as micrograms of retinol activity equivalents (mcg RAE) to account for both forms of the vitamin—retinol and carotenoids. Recommended intakes for people 14 years of age and older range from 700 to 900 mcg RAE per day. For pregnant women, recommended intakes range from 750 to 770 mcg RAE. Recommended intakes for nursing mothers range from 1,200 to 1,300 mcg RAE. Lower values are recommended for infants and children under age 14.

However, vitamin A is listed on most food and supplement labels in international units (IUs), not mcg RAE. The conversion rates between IU and mcg RAE are listed below:

1 IU RETINOL = 0.3 MCG RAE

1 IU BETA-CAROTENE FROM DIETARY SUPPLEMENTS = 0.15 MCG RAE

1 IU BETA-CAROTENE FROM FOOD = 0.05 MCG RAE

1 IU ALPHA-CAROTENE OR BETA-CRYPTOXANTHIN = 0.025 MCG RAE

For adults and children ages 4 and up, the FDA has established a vitamin A daily value (DV) of 5,000 IU from a varied diet of both plant and animal foods. DVs are not the same as recommended intakes. But trying to reach 100 percent of the DV each day will help ensure you're getting enough vitamin A.

Recommended Dietary Allowances (RDAs) for Vitamin A

LIFE STAGE GROUP	MCG OF RAE PER DAY
Infants 0–6 months	400 mcg RAE*
Infants 7–12 months	500 mcg RAE*
Children 1–3 years	300 mcg RAE
Children 4–8 years	400 mcg RAE
Children 9–13 years	600 mcg RAE
Teen boys 14–18 years	900 mcg RAE
Teen girls 14–18 years	700 mcg RAE
Men 19+ years	900 mcg RAE
Women 19+ years	700 mcg RAE
Pregnant teens 14–18 years	750 mcg RAE
Pregnant women 19+ years	770 mcg RAE
Breastfeeding teens 14–18 years	1,200 mcg RAE
Breastfeeding women 19+ years	1,300 mcg RAE

*Adequate Intake (AI)

Therapeutic Value of Vitamin A

In addition to treating deficiency syndromes, vitamin A has several potential preventive and therapeutic uses. Vitamin A is important medicine for the immune system. It keeps skin and mucous membrane cells healthy. When membranes are healthy they stay moist and resistant to cell damage. The moistness inhibits bacteria and viruses from "putting down stakes" and starting infectious diseases. Healthy cells are also resistant to cancers. Vitamin A fights cancer by inhibiting the production of DNA in cancerous cells. It slows down tumor growth in established cancers and may keep leukemia cells from dividing.

This vitamin is particularly helpful in diseases caused by viruses. Measles, respiratory viruses, and even human immunodeficiency virus (HIV), the virus that causes AIDS, may retreat in the presence of vitamin A. Blood levels of vitamin A are often low in people with viral illnesses. After receiving additional amounts of this vitamin, the body is able to mount its defenses, often resulting in a quicker recovery.

Carotenes like vitamin A support immune function, but in a different way. They stimulate the production of special white blood cells that help determine overall immune status. They improve the communication between cells, too, which results in fewer cell mutations. White blood cells attack bacteria, viruses, cancer cells, and yeast. Women with high levels of carotenes in their blood tend to have fewer incidences of vaginal yeast infections.

Deficiency of Vitamin A

Vitamin A deficiency is uncommon in the United States today, although it is still a common problem in many developing countries. Infants, young children, pregnant women, and breastfeeding women in developing countries are especially vulnerable.

The most common symptom of vitamin A deficiency in children and pregnant women is the eye condition xerophthalmia. One of the early signs of xerophthalmia is night blindness—the inability to see well in the dark. If the deficiency is not corrected, the outer layers of the eyes become dry, thickened, and cloudy, leading to blindness if left untreated.

Vitamin A deficiency also causes dry and rough skin, which can result in a kind of "goose flesh" appearance. In addition, this deficiency can cause one to become more susceptible to infectious diseases. That's because a lack of vitamin A damages the linings of the gastrointestinal and respiratory tracts; as a result, they can't act as effective barriers against bacteria. Infections of the vagina and the urinary tract are also more likely.

Vitamin A Excess

Large amounts of some forms of vitamin A can be harmful. Too much preformed vitamin A, or retinol, can cause dizziness, headaches, nausea, coma, and even death. High doses of preformed vitamin A (retinol) in pregnant women can also cause birth defects. Pregnant women should avoid high doses of vitamin A supplements.

Unlike preformed vitamin A, high intakes of beta-carotene or other forms of provitamin A is not known to be toxic. Consuming a lot of carotene-rich foods or taking high doses of beta-carotene supplements may turn your skin yellow-orange, but this condition is harmless.

The Tolerable Upper Intake Levels (ULs) for preformed vitamin A (retinol) are listed in the table on the next page. Upper limits for beta-carotene and other forms of provitamin A have not been established.

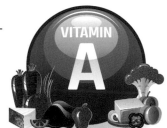

TOLERABLE UPPER INTAKE LEVELS (ULs) FOR PREFORMED VITAMIN A

LIFE STAGE GROUP	UPPER LIMIT
Infants 0–12 months	600 mcg RAE (2,000 IU)
Children 1–3 years	600 mcg RAE (2,000 IU)
Children 4–8 years	900 mcg RAE (3,000 IU)
Children 9–13 years	1,700 mcg RAE (5,667 IU)
Teens 14–18 years	2,800 mcg RAE (9,333 IU)
Adults 19+ years	3,000 mcg RAE (10,000 IU)
Pregnant and breastfeeding teens 14–18 years	2,800 mcg RAE (9,333 IU)
Pregnant and breastfeeding women 19+ years	3,000 mcg RAE (10,000 IU)

VITAMIN B6

Vitamin B$_6$ is the generic name for a group of water-soluble chemical compounds, including pyridoxine, pyridoxal, and pyridoxamine. The body needs vitamin B$_6$ for more than 100 enzyme reactions involved with metabolism.

Functions of Vitamin B6

Researchers discovered early on that vitamin B$_6$ was not one substance but three—pyridoxine, pyridoxal, and pyridoxamine. All three have the same biological activity and all three occur naturally in food.

Pyridoxine functions mainly by helping to metabolize protein and amino acids. Though not directly involved in the release of energy, like some other B vitamins, pyridoxine helps remove the nitrogen from amino acids, making them available as sources of energy. Because of its work with proteins, it plays a role in the synthesis of protein substances such as muscles, antibodies, and hormones. It also helps out in the production of red blood cells, neurotransmitters (chemical messengers), and prostaglandins that regulate certain metabolic processes. This vitamin gets together with more than 60 enzymes in the body, working to get many functions accomplished.

Pyridoxine

Pyridoxal

Pyridoxamine

Sources of Vitamin B6

Vitamin B_6 is in all foods, in one form or another. Plant foods are generally high in pyridoxine, while pyridoxamine and pyridoxal are more common in foods of animal origin. All three forms of vitamin B_6—pyridoxine, pyridoxamine, and pyridoxal—appear to have the same biological activity.

Protein foods, meats, whole wheat, salmon, nuts, wheat germ, brown rice, peas, and beans are good sources of vitamin B_6. Vegetables contain smaller amounts, but if eaten in large quantities, they can be an important source. Even though pyridoxine is lost when grains are milled to make flour, manufacturers do not regularly add it back to enriched products, except some highly fortified cereals.

The daily value (DV) for vitamin B_6 is 2 milligrams for adults and children ages 4 and up. However, the FDA does not require food labels to list vitamin B_6 content unless a food has been fortified with the nutrient.

Vitamin B_6 is also available in multivitamin-mineral supplements, in supplements containing B_6 with other B-complex vitamins, and as a standalone supplement. The most common form of vitamin B_6 in supplements is pyridoxine.

RECOMMENDED DIETARY ALLOWANCES (RDAs) FOR VITAMIN B6

LIFE STAGE GROUP	MILLIGRAMS PER DAY
Infants 0–6 months	0.1 mg*
Infants 7–12 months	0.3 mg*
Children 1–3 years	0.5 mg
Children 4–8 years	0.6 mg
Children 9–13 years	1.0 mg
Teen boys 14–18 years	1.3 mg
Teen girls 14–18 years	1.2 mg
Adults 19–50 years	1.3 mg
Men 51+ years	1.7 mg
Women 51+ years	1.5 mg
Pregnant teens and women	1.9 mg
Breastfeeding teens and women	2.0 mg

*Adequate Intake (AI)

Therapeutic Value of Vitamin B6

Entire books have been written on the therapeutic uses of vitamin B_6; it has been used to treat more than 100 health conditions.

Pyridoxine has a role in preventing heart disease. Without enough pyridoxine, a compound called homocysteine builds up in the body. Homocysteine damages blood vessel linings, setting the stage for plaque buildup when the body tries to heal the damage. Vitamin B_6 prevents this buildup, thereby reducing the risk of heart attack. Pyridoxine lowers blood pressure and blood cholesterol levels and keeps blood platelets from sticking together. All of these properties work to keep heart disease at bay.

Prone to kidney stones? Pyridoxine, teamed up with magnesium, prevents the formation of stones. It usually takes about three months of supplementation to make blood levels of these nutrients sufficient to keep stones from forming.

Vitamin B_6 has long been publicized as a cure for premenstrual syndrome (PMS). Some evidence suggests that vitamin B_6 supplements can ease PMS symptoms, including moodiness, irritability, forgetfulness, bloating, and anxiety. Vitamin B_6 supplements (in the form of pyridoxine) may also prevent premenstrual acne flare, a condition in which pimples break out about a week before a woman's period begins. Starting pyridoxine supplementation ten days before the menstrual period might prevent some pimples from forming. This effect is due to the vitamin's role in hormone regulation. Skin blemishes are typically caused by a hormone imbalance, which vitamin B_6 helps to regulate.

Depression is another condition that may result from low vitamin B_6 intake. Because of pyridoxine's role in serotonin and other neurotransmitter production, supplementation often helps depressed people feel better, and their mood improves significantly. It may also help improve memory in older adults. Women who are on hormone-replacement therapy or birth control pills often complain of depression and are frequently deficient in vitamin B_6. Supplementation improves these cases, too.

Low intakes of pyridoxine can slow down the immune system. Several different immune components become rather sluggish in the absence of adequate vitamin B_6, making a person more susceptible to diseases.

People with asthma can benefit from pyridoxine supplements. Clinical studies of the nutrient show that wheezing and asthma attacks decrease in severity and frequency during vitamin B_6 supplementation. Anyone with breathing difficulties who is taking the drug theophylline may want to consider supplementation with this vitamin. Theophylline interferes with vitamin B_6 metabolism. Supplementation not only normalizes blood levels but also helps limit the headaches, anxiety, and nausea that often accompany theophylline use.

The nausea and vomiting that frequently accompany the early stages of pregnancy sometimes respond to pyridoxine treatment.

Vitamin B6 Deficiency and Excess

Most people in the U.S. get enough vitamin B_6 from the foods in their diet. However, several groups of people are more likely to have low levels of vitamin B_6. These groups include people with kidney problems (such as those who are on kidney dialysis or have had a kidney transplant); people with autoimmune disorders (such as rheumatoid arthritis, celiac disease, Crohn's disease, ulcerative colitis, or inflammatory bowel disease); and people with alcohol dependence.

People with a vitamin B_6 deficiency can have a range of symptoms, including anemia, itchy rashes, scaly skin on the lips, cracks at the corners of the mouth, and a swollen tongue. Other symptoms of very low vitamin B_6 levels include depression, confusion, and a weak immune system. In infants, vitamin B_6 deficiency can cause irritability, extremely sensitive hearing, and seizures.

People almost never get too much vitamin B_6 from food sources. However, taking high doses of pyridoxine supplements for an extended period of time can cause severe nerve damage, leading people to lose control of their bodily movements. The symptoms usually disappear when the person stops taking the supplements. Other symptoms of too much vitamin B_6 include painful, unsightly skin patches, extreme sensitivity to sunlight, nausea, and heartburn.

VITAMIN B12

Vitamin B_{12} exists in several forms and contains the mineral cobalt. Vitamin B_{12} helps maintain healthy nerve and red blood cells, and is needed make DNA (the genetic material in all cells).

Vitamin B_{12} (also called cobalamin) is a water-soluble vitamin that plays essential roles in red blood cell formation, cell metabolism, nerve function, and the production of DNA (the genetic material in all cells).

Vitamin B_{12} differs from other vitamins, even those of the B complex, in many ways. The vitamin has a chemical structure much more complex than that of any other vitamin. It's the only vitamin to contain an inorganic element (cobalt) as an integral part of its makeup. Only microorganisms can make B_{12}. Plants and animals can't, although the vitamin does accumulate in animal products, which is where we get it.

A substance made in the stomach—called intrinsic factor—must be present to absorb vitamin B_{12} from the intestinal tract in significant amounts. Intrinsic factor combines with the vitamin B_{12} that is released from food during digestion. It carries the vitamin to the lower part of the small intestine, where, assisted by calcium, it attaches itself to special receptor cells. The vitamin B_{12} is then released from its carrier and enters these cells to be absorbed into the body. Without intrinsic factor, vitamin B_{12} misses its connection with the receptor cells and passes out of the body.

People with a condition known as pernicious anemia can't make intrinsic factor. As a result, they can't absorb vitamin B_{12}, even when there's plenty of the vitamin in their diets. Eventually, they show symptoms of a vitamin B_{12} deficiency. Pernicious anemia is a macrocytic, or large-cell, anemia similar to the anemia caused by folate deficiency.

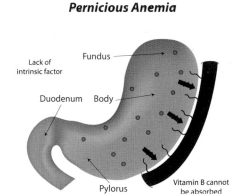

Pernicious Anemia

Lack of intrinsic factor

Fundus

Duodenum   Body

Pylorus

Vitamin B cannot be absorbed

History

The pursuit of vitamin B_{12} began in 1926 when two investigators found that patients who ate almost a pound of raw liver a day were effectively relieved of pernicious anemia. Scientists correctly speculated that liver contained a substance that prevents the disorder, but they wondered why victims of pernicious anemia needed so much of it. William B. Castle suggested that liver contained an antipernicious anemia (APA) factor. He also believed that people who had the disease lacked a factor intrinsically necessary to use the APA factor. By eating about a pound of liver a day, these people could counteract the lack of the intrinsic factor and absorb the APA factor they needed.

For the next 20 years, scientists searched for the APA factor. Progress was slow until 1948, when testing began on an experimental "animal"— the microorganism *Lactobacillus lactis*. Instead of testing liver extracts on people, researchers tested them on the microorganisms. Since these microorganisms reproduce so quickly, many generations could be tested in a short period of time. In less than a year, two research groups—one in England and one in the United States—both managed to isolate pure vitamin B_{12}.

Functions of Vitamin B12

Vitamin B_{12} is essential to cells because it's needed to make DNA (deoxyribonucleic acid) and RNA (ribonucleic acid), which carry and transmit genetic information for every living cell. This information tells a cell how to function and must be passed along each time a cell divides. Rapidly dividing cells need a continuous supply of vitamin B_{12}. This vitamin works along with the vitamin folate in this important role.

Vitamin B_{12} also helps maintain normal bone marrow. And it functions in the production of a material called myelin, which covers and protects nerve fibers. Vitamin B_{12} also plays a central role in folate metabolism. It releases free folate from its bound form so it can be absorbed, and it helps in the transportation and storage of folate. A deficiency of vitamin B_{12} can create a folate deficiency even when dietary intake of folate is adequate. That is why a deficiency of either vitamin causes a similar type of anemia.

Sources of Vitamin B12

Vitamin B_{12} is naturally found many animal foods, including beef liver, clams, fish, meat, poultry, eggs, milk, and other dairy products. Manufacturers also add vitamin B_{12} to some cereals and nutritional yeasts. Plant foods have no vitamin B_{12} unless they are fortified. Bacteria in the intestines make some vitamin B_{12}, but far less than the amount needed daily.

Vitamin B_{12} is also available in dietary supplements and in prescription medication. You can find the vitamin in almost all multivitamin-mineral supplements. It's also in supplements with other B vitamins and as a standalone supplement. Vitamin B_{12} is better absorbed when taken along with other B vitamins. You can also get vitamin B_{12} in a form that dissolves under your tongue. A prescription form of vitamin B_{12} can be given as a shot or as a nasal gel.

RECOMMENDED DIETARY ALLOWANCES (RDAs) FOR VITAMIN B12

LIFE STAGE GROUP	MICROGRAMS PER DAY
Infants 0–6 months	0.4 mcg*
Infants 7–12 months	0.5 mcg*
Children 1–3 years	0.9 mcg
Children 4–8 years	1.2 mcg
Children 9–13 years	1.8 mcg
Teens 14–18 years	2.4 mcg
Adults 19+ years	2.4 mcg
Pregnant teens and women	2.6 mcg
Breastfeeding teens and women	2.8 mcg

*Adequate Intake (AI)

Vitamin B12 Deficiency and Excess

When the supply of vitamin B_{12} in the body is low, it slows down the production of red blood cells (causing anemia) and the cells that line the intestine. This is similar to what happens as a result of insufficient folate. But unlike folate deficiency, a lack of vitamin B_{12} can also cause serious damage to the nervous system. If the condition persists for long, the damage is irreversible.

Most people in the U.S. get enough vitamin B_{12} from the foods they eat. However, some people have difficulty absorbing vitamin B_{12} from food. As a result, vitamin B_{12} deficiency is relatively common, affecting between 1.5 percent and 15 percent of the general public.

A deficiency of vitamin B_{12} caused by insufficient intake is not common. Dietary deficiency of vitamin B_{12} is usually seen only in strict vegetarians who don't eat foods of animal origin—not even milk or eggs.

Such a restricted diet is a particular problem for pregnant or breastfeeding women, since the baby can develop a vitamin B_{12} deficiency even if the mother remains healthy. For this reason, all vegetarian mothers should eat foods fortified with vitamin B_{12}. However, vegetarians who regularly eat eggs or drink milk get all the vitamin B_{12} they need.

Pernicious anemia is usually an inherited disease in which a deficiency of vitamin B_{12} occurs despite adequate amounts in the diet. People with this disease cannot produce intrinsic factor, the substance needed to absorb vitamin B_{12}. They need to receive injections of vitamin B_{12} so the vitamin can bypass the stomach and intrinsic factor and enter the bloodstream directly.

Pernicious anemia can also result from surgery. Because intrinsic factor originates in the stomach, partial or total removal of the stomach reduces absorption of vitamin B_{12}. Moreover, removal of the end of the small intestine (ileum) also creates a deficiency because that's where absorption of the vitamin takes place.

Stomach acid frees vitamin B_{12} from the proteins it is bound to in foods, but for the almost one half of adults who experience a decline in stomach acid as they age, this can be a problem. As many as 20 percent of people older than 65 may have low B_{12} blood levels. If undetected, the problem can cause nerve damage. An unexplained unsteady gait and loss of coordination are often the warning signs of this type of vitamin B_{12} deficiency.

There are no reports of vitamin B_{12} causing toxicity or adverse effects even when taken in large amounts. However, vitamin B_{12} can interact or interfere with several medicines. Talk to your health care provider before starting any dietary supplement.

VITAMIN C (ASCORBIC ACID)

When you hear the words vitamin C, you may instinctively think of the common cold. For that you can thank Linus Pauling (left) and his 1970 book, *Vitamin C and the Common Cold*. In it, Pauling recommended megadoses of vitamin C to reduce the frequency and severity of colds. The book triggered a sales boom for vitamin C that is still going strong. It also prompted nutritionists to begin a series of carefully designed studies of the vitamin and its functions.

Today, some people still swear by vitamin C. Researchers have found little proof of its effectiveness against catching the common cold, but there is evidence to suggest it can reduce the severity and length of a cold.

History

The story of vitamin C began centuries ago, with accounts of a disease called scurvy. The ailment causes muscle weakness, lethargy, poor wound healing, and bleeding from the gums and under the skin. Scurvy was rampant around the world for centuries. Ships' logs tell of its widespread occurrence among sailors in the 16th century.

Almost as old as reports of scurvy are reports of successful ways to treat the disease: eating green salads, fruits, vegetables, pickled cabbage, small onions, and an ale made of such things as wormwood, horseradish, and mustard seed. In the 1530s, French explorer Jacques Cartier (*left*) told how the natives of Newfoundland cured the mysterious disease by giving his men an extract prepared from the green shoots of an evergreen tree.

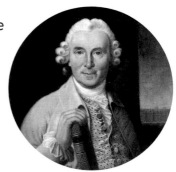

However, the disease was still the "scourge of the navy" until 1747 when British physician James Lind (*right*) singled out a cure for scurvy. Believing that acidic materials relieved symptoms of the illness, Lind tried six different substances on six groups of scurvy-stricken men.

He gave them all the standard shipboard diet, but to one pair of men in each of the six groups he gave a different test substance. One pair received a solution of sulfuric acid each day; another, cider; and a third, seawater. The fourth pair received vinegar, and the fifth took a daily combination of garlic, mustard seed, balsam of Peru, and gum myrrh. The sixth pair in the experiment received two oranges and a lemon each day.

Lind found that the men who ate citrus fruit improved rapidly; one returned to duty after only six days. The sailors who drank the cider showed slight improvement after two weeks, but none of the others improved.

Although Lind published the results of his experiment, decades passed before the British navy finally added lime juice to its sailors' diets, earning them the nicknames "limeys." And it wasn't until 1932 that researchers isolated the vitamin itself. At the time, it carried the name hexuronic acid. Later, scientists renamed it ascorbic (meaning "without scurvy") acid.

Functions of Vitamin C

A major function of vitamin C is its role as a cofactor in the formation and repair of collagen—the connective tissue that holds the body's cells and tissues together. Collagen is a primary component of blood vessels, skin, tendons, and ligaments. Vitamin C also promotes the normal development of bones and teeth. It's also needed for amino acid metabolism and the synthesis of hormones, including the thyroid hormone that controls the body's rate of metabolism. Vitamin C also aids the absorption of iron and calcium.

These days, vitamin C is heralded for its antioxidant status. It prevents other substances from combining with free oxygen radicals by tying up these free radicals of oxygen themselves. In this role, vitamin C protects a number of enzymes involved in functions ranging from cholesterol metabolism to immune function. It destroys harmful free radicals that damage cells and can lead to cancer, heart disease, cataracts, and perhaps even aging. Vitamin C rejuvenates its cousin antioxidant, vitamin E.

Sources of Vitamin C

Of course, the famed citrus fruits—oranges, lemons, grapefruits, and limes—are excellent sources of vitamin C. Other often overlooked excellent sources of vitamin C are strawberries, kiwifruit, cantaloupe, and peppers. Potatoes also supply vitamin C in significant amounts since they are widely consumed by Americans on a regular basis. Though cooking destroys some of the vitamin, you can minimize the amount lost if the temperature is not too high and you don't cook them any longer than necessary.

Rose hips from the rose plant—which are used to prepare rose-hip tea—are rich in vitamin C. Fruit juices, fruit juice drinks, and drink mixes may be fortified with vitamin C at fairly high levels.

More than any other vitamin except folate, vitamin C is easy to destroy. The amount of vitamin C in foods falls off rapidly during transport, processing, storage, and preparation. Bruising or cutting a fruit or vegetable destroys some of the vitamin, as do light, air, and heat. Still, if you cover and refrigerate orange juice, it will retain much of its vitamin C value, even after several days. For maximum vitamin value, it's best to use fresh, unprocessed fruits and vegetables whenever possible.

RECOMMENDED DIETARY ALLOWANCES (RDAs) FOR VITAMIN C

LIFE STAGE GROUP	MILLIGRAMS PER DAY
Infants 0–6 months	40 mg*
Infants 7–12 months	50 mg*
Children 1–3 years	15 mg
Children 4–8 years	25 mg
Children 9–13 years	45 mg
Teen boys 14–18 years	75 mg
Teen girls 14–18 years	65 mg
Men 19+ years	90 mg
Women 19+ years	75 mg
Pregnant teens 14–18 years	80 mg
Pregnant women 19+ years	85 mg
Breastfeeding teens 14–18 years	115 mg
Breastfeeding women 19+ years	120 mg
Smokers	Smokers require 35 mg/day more vitamin C than nonsmokers.

*Adequate Intake (AI)

Therapeutic Value of Vitamin C

Vitamin C is the most popular single vitamin supplement. Besides taking it to treat colds, people pop vitamin C capsules hoping that it will cure numerous ailments. There is now scientific evidence to support some of that hope.

Scientifically controlled studies using vitamin C for colds show that it can slightly reduce the severity of cold symptoms, acting as a natural antihistamine. The vitamin may be useful for allergy control for the same reason: It may reduce histamine levels. By giving the immune system one of the important nutrients it needs, extra vitamin C can often shorten the duration of the cold as well. However, studies have been unable to prove that megadoses of the vitamin can actually prevent the common cold.

As an important factor in collagen production, vitamin C is useful in wound healing of all types. From cuts and broken bones to burns and recovery from surgical wounds, vitamin C taken orally helps wounds to heal faster and better. Applied topically, vitamin C may protect the skin from free radical damage after exposure to ultraviolet (UV) rays.

Vitamin C makes the headlines when it comes to cancer prevention. Its antioxidant properties protect cells and their DNA from damage and mutation. It supports the body's immune system, the first line of defense against cancer, and prevents certain cancer-causing compounds from forming in the body. Vitamin C reduces the risk of getting almost all types of cancer. It appears that this nutrient doesn't directly attack cancer that has already occurred, but it helps keep the immune system nourished, enabling it to battle the cancer.

Vitamin C Deficiency and Excess

Vitamin C deficiency is rare in the U.S. today. However, people who get less than 10 milligrams of vitamin C per day for many weeks can get scurvy. People with scurvy can also develop anemia. Scurvy is fatal if left untreated. Fortunately, vitamin C supplements easily cure scurvy.

Taking too much vitamin C can cause diarrhea, nausea, and stomach upset. In people with a hereditary condition called hemochromatosis, which causes the body to store too much iron, chronic consumption of high doses of vitamin C could worsen iron overload and result in tissue damage.

VITAMIN D

Vitamin D is known as the sunshine vitamin for good reason. If you get enough sunshine, your body can make its own vitamin D. Vitamin D (also known as calciferol) is an essential nutrient for building and maintaining strong bones and teeth. It is a unique vitamin—your body can make its own vitamin D when sunlight makes contact with your skin. To get enough, it only takes a few minutes of sun exposure, three times a week, on your hands, arms, or face (without sunscreen). However, if you live in Northern climates or don't get outdoors much, especially in the winter, you shouldn't rely on sunshine. Also, as you age, your body may not be as efficient at making vitamin D, so food sources become even more important.

History

Years ago, few children in tropical countries developed the malformed bones and teeth characteristic of rickets. Yet many children in temperate climates and large industrial cities did. Why the difference? The sun.

Skin contains the substance provitamin D, which starts to convert to vitamin D when exposed to sunlight. In tropical countries, sunlight shone on children year-round. Since these children had ample opportunity for exposure, their skin formed adequate amounts of vitamin D, and thus they didn't experience the symptoms of rickets.

In the early 1900s, rickets afflicted large numbers of children in this country. While searching for the cause, researchers fed various diets to experimental animals. Those diets that prevented calcium from depositing in the bones produced the soft bones that are characteristic of rickets. From this research, investigators concluded that rickets was actually a vitamin-deficiency disease.

However, researchers were perplexed when they discovered that ultraviolet light could also prevent the deficiency. In the 1920s, nutritionists were able to prevent or cure rickets by feeding children cod liver oil or food exposed to ultraviolet light. They also prevented rickets by exposing children to direct sunlight or the light from a sunlamp. The explanation for these findings didn't crystallize for several more years. Cod liver oil was effective against rickets because it contains vitamin D. Foods exposed to ultraviolet light were effective because the light changed a substance in plant foods into a form of the vitamin that the body can use—vitamin D_2.

Today, doctors seldom see cases of rickets in the United States. The dramatic drop in rickets cases is primarily due to the increased availability of milk fortified with vitamin D.

Functions of Vitamin D

Vitamin D is necessary to help the body absorb the minerals calcium and phosphorus, which are needed for the proper growth and development of bones and teeth.

Whether it comes from food or is made in the skin, vitamin D must be activated before it's of use to the body. It first travels to the liver, where it undergoes a chemical change. Then it moves through the bloodstream to the kidneys, where it undergoes another change to become the active form of the vitamin. This active form—dihydroxy vitamin D—is the one that helps the body absorb calcium and phosphorus.

Sources of Vitamin D

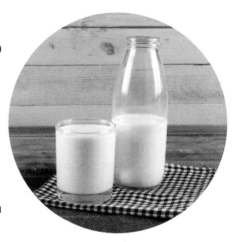

Your most reliable source of vitamin D is milk. Although milk is fortified with the vitamin, dairy products made from milk such as cheese, yogurt, and ice cream are generally not fortified with vitamin D. Only a few foods, including fatty fish (such as salmon, tuna, and mackerel) and fish oils, naturally contain significant amounts of vitamin D.

Other foods that contain smaller amounts of vitamin D include eggs, margarine, beef liver, and mushrooms, as well as fortified breakfast cereals, orange juice, yogurt, margarine, and soy beverages.

The vitamin D in supplements and fortified foods is found in two different forms: D_2 (ergocalciferol) and D_3 (cholecalciferol). Both increase vitamin D in the blood.

Recommended Intakes for Vitamin D

The RDAs for vitamin D represent a daily intake that is sufficient to maintain bone health and normal calcium metabolism in healthy people. RDAs for vitamin D are listed in both international units (IUs) and micrograms (mcg). These values are based on minimal sun exposure.

RECOMMENDED DIETARY ALLOWANCES (RDAs) FOR VITAMIN D

LIFE STAGE GROUP	RECOMMENDED AMOUNT
Infants 0–12 months	400 IU (10 mcg)*
Children 1–13 years	600 IU (15 mcg)
Teens 14–18 years	600 IU (15 mcg)
Adults 19–70 years	600 IU (15 mcg)
Adults 71+ years	800 IU (20 mcg)
Pregnant teens and women	600 IU (15 mcg)
Breastfeeding teens and women	600 IU (15 mcg)

*Adequate Intake (AI)

Deficiency of Vitamin D

People can become vitamin D deficient because they don't consume or absorb enough from food, their sunlight exposure is limited, or their kidneys cannot convert vitamin D to its active form in the body. In children, vitamin D deficiency causes rickets. Though rickets is rare in the United States today, some cases still occur, especially among African American infants and children. Vitamin D deficiency in adults leads to osteomalacia, which causes bone pain and muscle weakness.

Vitamin D Toxicity

Too much vitamin D can be toxic. As little as 3,000 IU a day can be toxic to children. Symptoms of overdose include diarrhea, nausea, vomiting, headache, weakness, weight loss, and elevated calcium levels in the blood. This condition, called hypercalcemia, can lead to calcium deposits in the kidneys, heart, and other tissues, causing irreversible damage. Excessive sun exposure does not result in vitamin D toxicity because the body limits the amount of this vitamin it produces.

VITAMIN E

Vitamin E is not a single compound, but several different compounds, all with vitamin E activity. One, alpha-tocopherol (or α-tocopherol), has the greatest activity. Other compounds with vitamin E activity are beta-tocopherol, gamma-tocopherol, and delta-tocopherol.

Functions of Vitamin E

Vitamin E functions as an antioxidant in the cells and tissues of the body. It protects polyunsaturated fats and other oxygen-sensitive compounds such as vitamin A from being destroyed by damaging oxidation reactions.

Vitamin E's antioxidant properties are also important to cell membranes. For example, vitamin E protects lung cells that are in constant contact with oxygen and white blood cells that help fight disease. A deficiency of vitamin E thus weakens the immune system.

But the benefits of vitamin E's antioxidant role may go much further. Vitamin E may protect against heart disease and may slow the deterioration associated with aging. Critics scoffed at such claims in the past, but an understanding of the importance of vitamin E's antioxidant role may be beginning to pay off.

Sources of Vitamin E

Oils and margarines from corn, cottonseed, soybean, safflower, and wheat germ are all good sources of vitamin E. Generally, the more polyunsaturated oil is, the more vitamin E it contains, serving as its own built-in protection. Fruits, vegetables, and whole grains have smaller amounts. Refining grains reduces their vitamin E content, as does commercial processing and storage of food. Cooking foods at high temperatures also destroys vitamin E, so a polyunsaturated oil is useless as a vitamin E source if it's used for frying. Your best sources are fresh and lightly processed foods, as well as those that aren't overcooked.

These days, it's difficult to get much vitamin E in the diet because of cooking and processing losses and because of the generally reduced intake of fat. Moreover, the current emphasis on monounsaturated fats, such as olive oil or canola oil, rather than vitamin E-containing polyunsaturated fats, further decreases our intake of vitamin E. Monounsaturated fats have other benefits for the heart, though, so you shouldn't stop using olive and canola oils. It is important to find other sources of vitamin E. Besides, the fewer polyunsaturated fats you eat, the less vitamin E you need, so your requirements may be lower if you switch to olive or canola oils.

Vitamin E from natural sources is usually listed on food packaging and supplement labels as "d-alpha-tocopherol" or "D-alpha-tocopherol." Synthetic vitamin E is usually listed as "dl-alpha-tocopherol" or "DL-alpha-tocopherol." The synthetic form of vitamin E is only half as active as the natural form.

Most once-a-day multivitamin-mineral supplements provide about 30 IU of vitamin E (the daily value), whereas standalone vitamin E supplements usually contain 100 to 1,000 IU per pill—much higher than the recommended amounts. Daily use of large-dose vitamin E supplements (400 IU/day) may increase the risk of prostate cancer.

Recommended Intakes for Vitamin E

The RDAs for vitamin E in the table below are given in milligrams (mg) and in international units (IU). Labels on foods and dietary supplements have typically listed the amount of vitamin E in IU. However, under the FDA's new labeling regulations, vitamin E will be listed only in milligrams (mg). These values are for the natural form of alpha-tocopherol.

RECOMMENDED DIETARY ALLOWANCES (RDAs) FOR VITAMIN E (NATURAL FORM OF ALPHA-TOCOPHEROL)

LIFE STAGE GROUP	RECOMMENDED AMOUNT
Infants 0–6 months	4 mg (6 IU)*
Infants 7–12 months	5 mg (7.5 IU)*
Children 1–3 years	6 mg (9 IU)
Children 4–8 years	7 mg (10.4 IU)
Children 9–13 years	11 mg (16.4 IU)
Teens 14–18 years	15 mg (22.4 IU)
Adults 19+ years	15 mg (22.4 IU)
Pregnant teens and women	15 mg (22.4 IU)
Breastfeeding teens and women	19 mg (28.4 IU)

*Adequate Intake (AI)

Vitamin E Deficiency and Excess

No obvious symptoms accompany a vitamin E deficiency, making it hard to detect. A brownish pigmentation of the skin may signal the problem, but only a blood test can confirm if vitamin E levels are actually too low. When diseases of the liver, gallbladder, or pancreas reduce intestinal absorption, a mild deficiency of vitamin E can result. A diet of processed foods that's very low in fat might also cause a deficiency.

Eating vitamin E in foods is not harmful. However, high doses of vitamin E in supplements can delay blood clotting, possibly causing an increased risk of stroke or uncontrolled bleeding in the event of an accident. Because of this possibility, people on anticoagulant therapy (blood thinners) should not take large doses of vitamin E.

Adults should take no more than 1,500 IU per day for supplements made from the natural form or 1,100 IU per day from supplements made from the synthetic form of vitamin E. The upper limits for children are lower than those for adults.

VITAMIN K

Vitamin K is the generic name for a family of compounds with a common chemical structure. These include phylloquinone (vitamin K_1), menaquinone (vitamin K_2), and menadione (vitamin K_3).

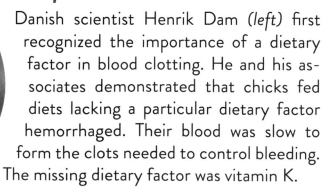

History

Danish scientist Henrik Dam *(left)* first recognized the importance of a dietary factor in blood clotting. He and his associates demonstrated that chicks fed diets lacking a particular dietary factor hemorrhaged. Their blood was slow to form the clots needed to control bleeding. The missing dietary factor was vitamin K.

Functions of Vitamin K

Vitamin K plays an important role in forming blood clots and maintaining strong bones, and also has other functions in the body. The proteins used in blood clotting require vitamin K. When there isn't enough of the vitamin, blood takes longer to clot, which can increase the amount of blood lost. Vitamin K also helps make a protein that may help regulate blood calcium levels. Calcium, usually associated with keeping bones strong, is also necessary for blood clotting.

Sources of Vitamin K

Food sources of vitamin K include green leafy vegetables (such as kale, spinach, broccoli, and lettuce), vegetable oils (such as soybean and canola oil), some fruits (such as blueberries and figs), meat, cheese, eggs, and soybeans. The best food sources of phylloquinone (vitamin K_1) are green leafy vegetables (especially collards, turnip greens, spinach, kale, parsley, and broccoli), pumpkin, okra, soybean oil, carrot juice, pomegranate juice, and prunes. Meat, dairy products, and eggs contain low levels of phylloquinone but modest amounts of menaquinones (vitamin K_2).

We get some of the vitamin K we need from the foods we eat. The rest comes from the bacteria that live in our digestive tracts and produce vitamin K. The extent to which we are able to use bacterially produced vitamin K, however, is still somewhat uncertain.

Vitamin K is also available as a dietary supplement. Vitamin K is found in multivitamin-mineral supplements, in standalone supplements, and in supplements with other nutrients, frequently calcium, magnesium, and/or vitamin D. Several forms of vitamin K are used in dietary supplements, in-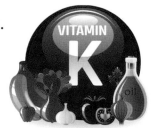cluding vitamin K_1 as phylloquinone or phytonadione (a synthetic form of vitamin K_1) and vitamin K_2 as menaquinone-4 (MK-4) or menaquinone-7 (MK-7).

Recommended Intakes for Vitamin K

There was insufficient data available to establish RDAs for vitamin K, so adequate intakes (AIs) for all ages were established instead. The current AIs are listed in micrograms (mcg).

ADEQUATE INTAKES (AIs) FOR VITAMIN K

LIFE STAGE GROUP	MICROGRAMS PER DAY
Infants 0–6 months	2.0 mcg
Infants 7–12 months	2.5 mcg
Children 1–3 years	30 mcg
Children 4–8 years	55 mcg
Children 9–13 years	60 mcg
Teens 14–18 years	75 mcg
Men 19+ years	120 mcg
Women 19+ years	90 mcg
Pregnant and breastfeeding teens 14–18 years	75 mcg
Pregnant and breastfeeding women 19+ years	90 mcg

Vitamin K Deficiency and Excess

Most people in the United States get enough vitamin K from the foods they eat and from the vitamin K made by bacteria in the colon. Significant vitamin K deficiency is very rare in adults. It is usually limited to people with malabsorption disorders (such as cystic fibrosis, celiac disease, ulcerative colitis, and short bowel syndrome) or those taking drugs that interfere with vitamin K metabolism.

Newborn babies, especially those born prematurely, are born with little vitamin K. For the first couple of days after birth, the baby's intestinal tract has no bacteria to make the vitamin either. Because the lack of vitamin K could lead to bleeding problems, newborns are routinely given a vitamin K injection.

Vitamin K consumption from food or supplements has not been shown to cause any harm. However, it can interact with some medications, particularly anticoagulants (blood thinners, such as warfarin).

ZEAXANTHIN

Zeaxanthin is a substance found in foods that are bright yellow, orange and green. It is a carotenoid the body cannot use to make vitamin A. Along with lutein, this pigment in the carotenoid family is linked to a reduced risk of age-related macular degeneration and cataracts. Good food sources of zeaxanthin include corn, leafy green vegetables, persimmons, tangerines, seeds, and egg yolk.

ZINC

Most zinc resides in our bones. The rest of this trace mineral turns up in skin, hair, and nails. In men, the prostate gland contains more zinc than any other organ.

Functions of Zinc

Zinc is a part of more than 200 different enzyme systems that aid the metabolism of carbohydrates, fats, and proteins. One of these enzymes, superoxide dismutase, serves as an antioxidant in cells. Zinc is also part of the hormone insulin, helping transport vitamin A from its storage site in the liver to where it is used in the body.

Sources of Zinc

Oysters contain more zinc than any other food. Meat, poultry, seafood, eggs, liver, and fortified breakfast cereals are also rich sources. Beans, nuts, dairy products, and whole grains provide some zinc. Two servings of animal protein daily provide most of the zinc a healthy person needs. Whole grains contain fair amounts of zinc, but they also harbor 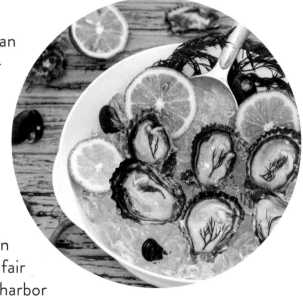 phytates, substances that tie up zinc and other minerals and prevent absorption. Yeast counteracts the action of phytates, so eating whole-grain breads still affords good nutrition.

Zinc is found in almost all multivitamin-mineral supplements. It is also available in dietary supplements containing only zinc or combined with calcium, magnesium, or other ingredients. Dietary supplements can have several different forms of zinc including zinc gluconate, zinc sulfate, and zinc acetate.

RECOMMENDED DIETARY ALLOWANCES (RDAs) FOR ZINC

LIFE STAGE GROUP	MILLIGRAMS PER DAY
Infants 0–6 months	2 mg*
Infants 7–12 months	3 mg
Children 1–3 years	3 mg
Children 4–8 years	5 mg
Children 9–13 years	8 mg
Teen boys 14–18 years	11 mg
Teen girls 14–18 years	9 mg
Men 19+ years	11 mg
Women 19+ years	8 mg
Pregnant teens 14–18 years	12 mg
Pregnant women 19+ years	11 mg
Breastfeeding teens 14–18 years	13 mg
Breastfeeding women 19+ years	12 mg

*Adequate Intake (AI)

Therapeutic Value of Zinc

Optimal immune function is vital for avoiding colds, flu, cancer, and infectious diseases in general. Zinc supplements before and during an illness can help the body put up a better fight. Zinc lozenges dissolved slowly in the mouth help to resolve a cold and sore throat. Viruses responsible for illness are inhibited by zinc; they're unable to replicate.

Zinc Deficiency and Excess

Zinc deficiency is rare in North America. When it does occur, zinc deficiency has serious effects, including retarded growth and sexual development, delayed wound healing, a low sperm count, depressed immune system (making infections more likely), reduced appetite, and altered sense of taste and smell.

As with other minerals, taking too much zinc can have the opposite of the effect desired. Excessive amounts will depress immune function and create other deficiencies and complications, such as skin outbreaks, high blood cholesterol levels, anemia, and scurvy-like symptoms. Excess zinc can also cause a copper deficiency.